COFFEE, CHOCOLATE, TEA, SODA REPLACED

COFFEE, CHOCOLATE, TEA, SODA REPLACED

Frederick Mickel Huck

authorHOUSE®

AuthorHouse™ LLC
1663 Liberty Drive
Bloomington, IN 47403
www.authorhouse.com
Phone: 1-800-839-8640

Published by AuthorHouse   11/22/2013

ISBN: 978-1-4918-2684-3 (sc)
ISBN: 978-1-4918-2683-6 (e)

CONTENTS

This book is dedicated to:

ROBERT E MENZIE
INEZ A MENZIE
DONALD W HUCK
AURA V HUCK
DR EDE KOENIG

Special thanks to:

Sandra V Mooney
Matthew F Mooney
John Dunlap
Angie Ingersoll

SOME FACTS ON COFFEE

Each day approximately fifty million gallons of coffee is consumed in the United States. Coffee is high in caffeine which stimulates the heart, by increasing the heart rate, and can cause irregular heartbeats. Coffee is addictive, increases your appetite, and has no nutritional value. It raises blood cholesterol, reduces blood supply, causes sleep disturbances, fatigue, dehydration, and memory loss. It removes calcium, produces headaches, causes stress in the pancreas, increases recklessness, hostility, and anxiety. Coffee increases cancer in the bladder, lungs, kidneys, stomach, ovarian, colon, and prostate. It can promote eating disorders. Some of the symptoms are out right noticeable, while others take longer to be discovered. Replacing coffee was very easy. The product is Roma a natural combination of roasted malt barley, roasted barley and roasted chicory. There are numerous recipes, which utilize Roma. Cakes, pies, cookies, candy, coated roasted nuts, frostings, ice cream, etc. You can also drink it.

SOME FACTS ABOUT CHOCOLATE

The cocoa tree grows in the tropical areas of our planet. The beans come in pods and they are heated and into finely grind into a powder and are very bitter. Chocolate also contains the following: caffeine, theo bromine, theophylline, and tannin, oxalic acid. fermentation, sugar, oils, milk, animal fat, rodent hairs (powder), insect parts, (fragments), mold, and bacteria.

Chocolate has side effects: cancer of the digestive tract and other digestive disorders, depression and anxiety, calcium deficiencies, chemical toxicity, allergies, and more. Chocolate in any form does not belong in your body. It is also not natural due to all the additives and preservatives to make it palatable. It goes through harsh over processing.

There is no known nutritional value for the body. However, carob is a very good replacement for chocolate. After some processing, the chocolate is sold in a form of powder. I have over seventy-five recipes, which contain carob, cakes, pies, cookies, candy, fudges, covered nuts, frostings, ice creams, etc. Carob can also be mixed with soymilk. Carob contains protein fiber, is low in fat, contains B vitamins, calcium, magnesium, iron, potassium, pectin, manganese, chromium, copper, and nickel. Carob is also used for relieving nausea, diarrhea, vomiting; it is good for the stomach and intestinal lining.

CAFFEINE

Caffeine can be found in coffee, chocolate, tea, and sodas; and is mind altering and addictive. It irritates the kidneys, creates problems in sleep; therefore causes fatigue and lack of energy. Caffeine will cause disease including a lowered immune system and bone problems. Quitting its use will cause withdrawal symptoms, this alone should verify that caffeine does not belong in your body. Sodas, diet or regular containing caffeine can also alter ones sleeping habits. The added sugars or sugar substitutes plus sodium are other factors to stop drinking sodas.

GUIDE 14 DAYS

The purpose of this fourteen day meal plan is to illustrate that starvation does not exist when following the plan. Instead of listing the fruit on a daily log every day, I just list here approximately, what was eaten.

For the last two years, I have reversed my two meals. The larger was consumed first and the second is mostly raw. Prior to eating breakfast, generally a half an hour after I wake, I drink a quart of warm water with two teaspoons of lemon juice, one tablespoon of inland sea water and one tablespoon of silver mineral water. I consume approximately five pounds of fruit daily, and the fruit varies according to the seasons of the year.

The fourteen days are very similar (fruit meal) and they are three different colors of apples, twelve cherries, one nectarine, one mango, one slice of pineapple, one slice of cantaloupe, eight green grapes, one apricot, and one peach. In addition I also, eat eight raw Brazil nuts, 6 apricot nuts, one teaspoon of sunflower seeds, and one teaspoon of pumpkin seeds, two capsules of calcium, two capsules of magnesium.

For dinner, I usually have a salad, which consists of red or green head lettuce three radishes cut small one long green, onion cut small one third of a carrot, cut small one-half of avocado one-half of celery stalk cut small six tablespoons of lemon juice approximately one tablespoon or more of Braggs Ammino up to twelve ounces or more of two different kinds of Hot Sauce bread, or crackers, or corn tortillas

Please do not copy or give away any material, not just, because it is copyright protected material, but doing this will interfere with my program of feeding and educating the unhealthy. All book proceeds as of 2008 have gone into this program. Instead my wish is that you do share your cooking with friends, family, and strangers.

Questions, concerns, and suggestions are welcome:

7619 N "8th" St
Fresno, CA 93720-2644
Phone 559 435 4069

14 DAYS OF MEALS

Day 1

Breakfast: Raw Nut Mix Combination, fresh fruit,
              Pumpkin seed waffles

Dinner: Salad, Crackers, Vegetable soup

Dessert: Cinnamon Ice Cream

Notes   _____

         _____

         _____

Day 2

Breakfast: Raw nut mix combination. Fresh fruit
             Cajun dried roasted nut mix

Dinner: Salad, Lavish-Tonir bread, Tamales
             Spanish rice

Dessert: Brazil Nut Fudge

Notes   _____
             _____
             _____

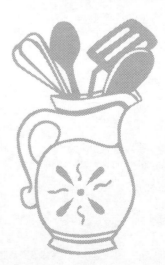

Day 3

Breakfast: Raw nut mix combination, fresh fruit
              Havenero Rice

Dinner: Salad, corn tortillas
              Tomato casserole

Dessert: Plum Tofu cookies

Notes   _____
              _____
              _____

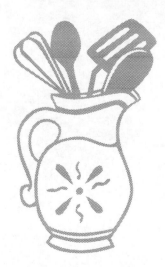

Day 4

Breakfast: Raw nut mix combination, fresh fruit
Popcorn

Dinner: Salad. Garlic Bread, Pasta

Dessert: Peppermint Salt Water Taffy

Notes   _____
_____
_____

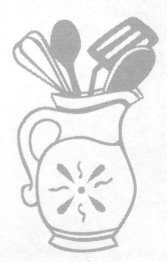

Day 5

Breakfast: Raw nut mix combination, fresh fruit
             Bell Pepper Rice

Dinner: Salad, Bean burrito

Dessert: Peach Cream Pie

Notes   _____
             _____
             _____

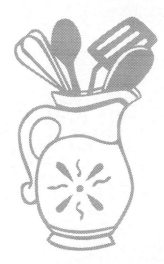

Day 6

Breakfast: Raw nut mix combination, fresh fruit
              Cajun Rice

Dinner: Salad, Egg rolls

Dessert: Maple Syrup cookies

Notes   _____
              _____
              _____

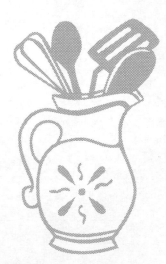

Day 7

Breakfast: Raw nut mix combination, fresh fruit
            Lemon Garlic rice

Dinner: Salad, crackers, deep dish pizza

Dessert: Pecan candy

Notes   _____
            _____
            _____

Day 8

Breakfast: Raw nut mix combination, fresh fruit
             Cashew waffles

Dinner: Taco Salad, Lavish-tonir Bread

Dessert: Carob cake

Notes   _____
             _____
             _____

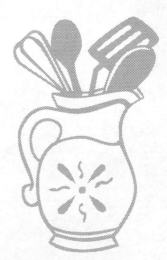

Day 9

Breakfast: Raw nut mix combination, fresh fruit
             Walnut waffles

Dinner: Salad, Garlic Bread, Lentils, and baked rice

Dessert: Plum cup cookies

Notes   _____
             _____
             _____

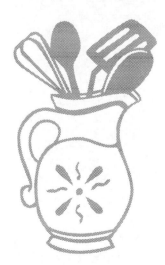

Day 10

Breakfast: Raw nut mix combination, fresh fruit
            Pigeon Rice

Dinner: Salad, crackers, enchiladas

Dessert: Carob macaroons

Notes   _____
            _____
            _____

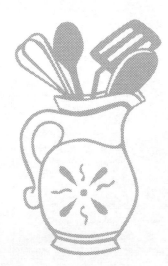

Day 11

Breakfast: Raw nut mix combination, fresh fruit
             Pancakes

Dinner: Salad, Lavish tonir bread
             Black eye pea rice

Dessert: Walnut pie

Notes   _____
             _____
             _____

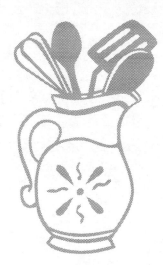

Day 12

Breakfast: Raw nut mix combination, fresh fruit
            Pancakes

Dinner: Salad, garlic toast, pot pie

Dessert: Carob pie

Notes   _____

            _____

            _____

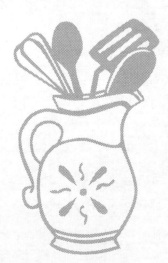

Day 13

Breakfast: Raw nut mix combination, fresh fruit
             Green Pepper rice

Dinner: Crackers, salad,
             Stuffed bell peppers

Dessert: Date cookies

Notes   _____

             _____

             _____

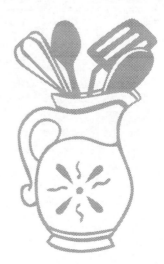

Day 14

Breakfast: Raw nut mix combination, fresh fruit
              Toast with Cherry jam

Dinner: Salad, Lavish tonir bread, Chinese Pan Fried Noodles
              Chinese rice

Dessert: Roma dried roasted nut mix

Notes   _____
              _____
              _____

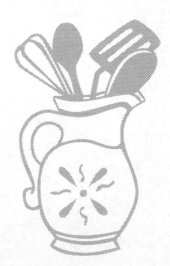

Recipe 443

Vanilla Cake Frosting

Place in a vitamix the following:

6 cup of sucanant sugar (3 cups at a time)
make into a fine powder.

Pour into a bowl and mix the following:
3 tablespoons of maple syrup

Mix and add
2 tablespoons of Vanilla
then add 3 tablespoons of water—(add one tablespoon of water at a time)

this will make mixture thinner.

Place frosting on cake when cake is cold.
Return cake to refrigerator.

Serve cold

Notes _____

_____

_____

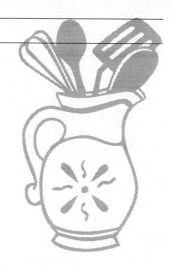

Peach Maple Cake

Place into vitamix the following:

2 peaches (remove seed/stem)
1 Tablespoon of Biosalt
2 Tablespoons of Almond Butter
1 teaspoon of vanilla
6 cups of maple syrup

Mix and pour into a large bowl and add:

6 cups of grinded walnuts
4 cups of sifted whole wheat pastry flour

Mix and pour into glass dish 9 x 13 inches lined with parchment paper.
Bake 350 degrees for 90 minutes.
Check every 10 minutes after 60 minutes . . . use toothpick test to see if center
    is done.

Notes   _____

_____

_____

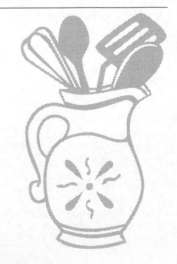

Plum Maple Cake

Place into vitamix the following:

2 cups of plums (remove seeds only)
1 Tablespoon of Biosalt
2 Tablespoons of Almond Butter
1 teaspoon of vanilla
6 cups of maple syrup

Mix and pour into a large bowl and add:

6 cups of grinded walnuts
4 cups of sifted whole wheat pastry flour

Mix and pour into glass dish 9 x 13 inches lined with parchment paper.
Bake 350 degrees for 90 minutes.
Check every 10 minutes after one hour . . . use toothpick test to see if center
    is baked

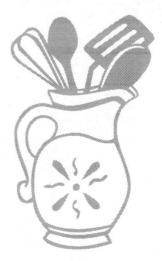

Recipe 446

Apricot Maple Cake

Place into vitamix the following:

2 cups of Apricots (remove seed only)
1 Tablespoon of Biosalt
2 Tablespoons of Almond Butter
1 teaspoon of vanilla
6 cups of maple syrup

Mix and pour into a large bowl and add:

6 cups of grinded walnuts
4 cups of sifted whole wheat pastry flour

Mix and pour into glass dish 9 x 13 inches lined with parchment paper.
Bake 350 degrees 90 minutes.
Check every 10 minutes after 60 minutes . . . use toothpick test to see if center
   is baked

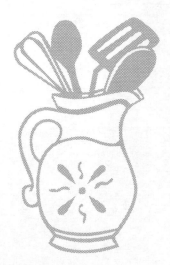

Recipe 447

Pineapple Maple Cake

Place into vitamix thc following:

2 cups of Pineapple
1 Tablespoon of Biosalt
2 Tablespoons of Almond Butter
1 teaspoon of vanilla
6 cups of maple syrup

Mix and pour into a large bowl and ad:

6 cups of grinded walnuts
4 cups of sifted whole wheat pastry flour

Mix and pour into glass dish 9 x 13 inches lined with parchment paper.
Bake 350 degrees for 90 minutes.
Check every 10 minutes after 60 minutes . . . use toothpick test to see if center
    is baked

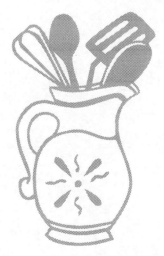

Recipe 448

Apple Maple Cake

Place into vitamix the following:

2 large apples or 4 small (remove core only)
1 Tablespoon of Biosalt
2 Tablespoons of Almond Butter
1 teaspoon of vanilla
6 cups of maple syrup

Mix and pour into a large bowl and add:

6 cups of grinded walnuts
4 cups of sifted whole wheat pastry flour

Mix and pour into glass dish 9 x 13 inches lined with parchment paper.
Bake 350 degrees for 90 minutes.
Check every 10 minutes after 60 minutes . . . use toothpick test to see if center is
    baked.

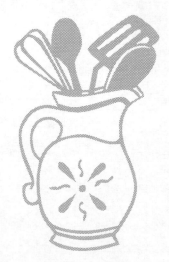

Recipe 449

Cherry Maple Cake

Place into vitamix the following:

2 cups of cherries (remove seeds/stem)
1 Tablespoon of Biosalt
2 Tablespoons of Almond Butter
1 teaspoon of vanilla
6 cups of maple syrup

Mix and pour into a large bowl and add:

6 cups of grinded walnuts
4 cups of sifted whole wheat pastry flour

Mix and pour into glass dish 9 x 13 inches lined with parchment paper.
Bake 350 degrees for 90 minutes.
Check every 10 minutes after 60 minutes . . . use toothpick test to see if center
    is baked

Recipe 450

Nectarine Maple Cake

Place into vitamix the following:

2 cups of Nectarines
1 Tablespoon of Biosalt
2 Tablespoons of Almond Butter
1 teaspoon of vanilla
6 cups of maple syrup

Mix and pour into a large bowl and add:

6 cups of grinded walnuts
4 cups of sifted whole wheat pastry flour

Mix and pour into glass dish 9 x 13 inches lined with parchment paper.
Bake 350 degrees for 90 minutes.
Check every 10 minutes after 60 minutes . . . use toothpick test to see if center is
    baked.

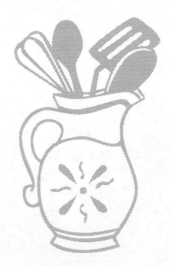

Recipe 451

Lemon Maple Cake

Place into vitamix the following:

1 cup of lemon rind and 1 cup of lemon juice
1 Tablespoon of Biosalt
2 Tablespoons of Almond Butter
1 teaspoon of vanilla
6 cups of maple syrup

Mix and pour into a large bowl and add:

6 cups of grinded walnuts
4 cups of sifted whole wheat pastry flour

Mix and pour into glass dish 9 x 13 inches lined with parchment paper.
Bake 350 degrees for 90 minutes.
Check every 10 minutes after 60 minutes . . . use toothpick test to see if center
   is baked

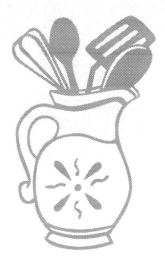

Recipe 452

Orange Maple Cake

Place into vitamix the following:

2 cups of Orange juice or 1 cup of orange juice and 1 cup of Orange Rind
1 Tablespoon of Biosalt
2 Tablespoons of Almond Butter
1 teaspoon of vanilla
6 cups of maple syrup

Mix and pour into a large bowl and add:

6 cups of grinded walnuts
4 cups of sifted whole wheat pastry flour

Mix and pour into glass dish 9 x 13 inches lined with parchment paper.
Bake 350 degrees for 90 minutes.
Check every 10 minutes after 60 minutes . . . use toothpick test to see if center is
    baked.

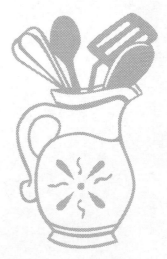

Recipe 453

Blueberry Maple Cake

Place into vitamix the following:

2 cups of Blueberries
1 Tablespoon of Biosalt
2 Tablespoons of Almond Butter
1 teaspoon of vanilla
6 cups of maple syrup

Mix and pour into a large bowl and add:

6 cups of grinded walnuts
4 cups of sifted whole wheat pastry flour

Mix and pour into glass dish 9 x 13 inches lined with parchment paper.
Bake 350 degrees for 90 minutes.
Check every 10 minutes after 60 minutes . . . use toothpick test to see if center is
    baked.

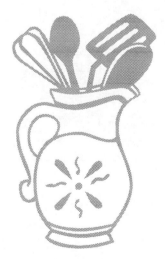

Recipe 454

Pear Maple Cake

Place into vitamix the following:

2 cups of pears or 2 large pears.
1 Tablespoon of Biosalt
2 Tablespoons of Almond Butter
1 teaspoon of vanilla
6 cups of maple syrup

Mix and pour into a large bowl and add:

6 cups of grinded walnuts
4 cups of sifted whole wheat pastry flour

Mix and pour into glass dish 9 x 13 inches lined with parchment paper.
Bake 350 degrees for 90 minutes.
Check every 10 minutes after 50 minutes . . . use toothpick test to see if center is
    baked.

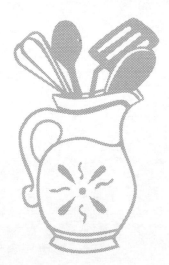

Recipe 455

Blueberry Baked Alaska

Place in a vitamix

1 cup of sucanant sugar
1 cup of maple syrup
1 cup of almond butter
One half cup of Blueberries
1 Brick or one pound of Tofu

Mix and place into four baking dishes
I use the same dishes for pot pies 7 x 7 inches
Bake 350 degrees 20 minutes
Let Cool serve cold or semi frozen
Freeze extra covered

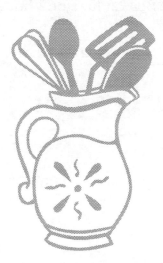

Recipe 456

Bar B Que Hot Sauce

Place the following into Vitamix:
26 to 31 Tomatoes
4 cups of water
1 cup of maple syrup
2 cups of lemon juice
1 cup of cilantro
1 cup of Braggs
2 bell peppers
8-12 Haverero peppers
8 cloves of garlic
4 stalks of celery
1 large onion
4 tablespoons of paprika
4 tablespoons of chili powder
2 tablespoons of Biosalt
1 tablespoon of cumin
1 tablespoon of turmeric
1 tablespoon of clove powder
1 tablespoon of ginger powder

Boil on low for 2 hours or more until sauce is thick

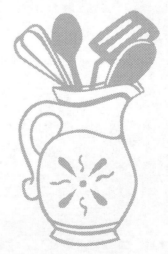

Recipe 457

Pistachio Waffles

Place following into a vitamix

6 cups of soymilk or water
4 cups of oatmeal
1 cup of pistachios
2 teaspoons of Biosalt
one half cup of sesame seeds or almond butter

Mix and pour into waffle iron one spoon at a time—spread even cook 13-15
    minutes
Let waffle cool
Freeze extra
when ready to rewarm place in a toaster oven

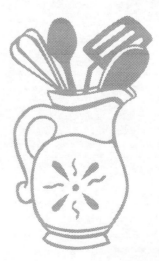

Recipe 458

Peach Baked Alaska

Place in a vitamix

1 cup of sucanant sugar
1 cup of maple syrup
1 cup of almond butter
One peach or one cup (remove stem & seed to make one cup)
1 Brick or one pound of Tofu

Mix and place into baking dishes 4 dishes needed
I use the same dishes for pot pies 7 x 7 inches
Bake 350 degrees 20 minutes
Let Cool serve cold or semi frozen
Freeze extra covered

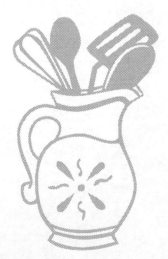

Recipe 459

Apricot Baked Alaska

Place following in a vitamix

1 cup of sucanant sugar
1 cup of maple sugar
1 cup of Apricots (remove pits only)
1 brick or one pound of tofu
1 cup almond butter

Mix until very smooth
pour mixture into baking dishes 4 to 5 needed
I use same dishes for pot pies 7 x 7 inches
Bake 350 degrees 20 minutes
Let Cool serve cold or semi frozen
Freeze extra covered

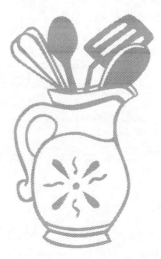

Recipe 460

Apple Baked Alaska

Place in a vitamix

1 cup of sucanant sugar
1 cup of maple syrup
1 cup of almond butter
One cup or one large apple (remove core)
1 Brick or one pound of Tofu

Mix and place into baking dishes 4 dishes needed
I use the same dishes for pot pies 7 x 7 inches
Bake 350 degrees 20 minutes
Let Cool serve cold or semi frozen
Freeze extra covered

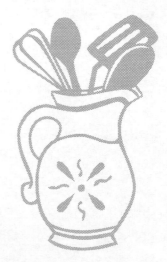

Recipe 461

Plum Baked Alaska

Place in a vitamix

1 cup of sucanant sugar
1 cup of maple syrup
1 cup of almond butter
One cup of plums (remove seed/stem only)
1 Brick or one pound of Tofu

Mix and place into baking dishes 4 dishes needed
I use the same dishes for pot pies 7 x 7 inches
Bake 350 degrees 20 minutes
Let Cool serve cold or semi frozen
Freeze extra covered

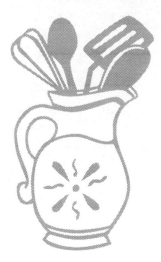

Recipe 462

Nectarine Baked Alaska

Place in a vitamix

1 cup of sucanant sugar
1 cup of maple syrup
1 cup of almond butter
One cup of nectarine or one large nectarine (remove seed only)
1 Brick or one pound of Tofu

Mix and place into baking dishes 4 dishes needed
I use the same dishes for pot pies 7 x 7 inches
Bake 350 degrees 20 minutes
Let Cool serve cold or semi frozen
Freeze extra covered

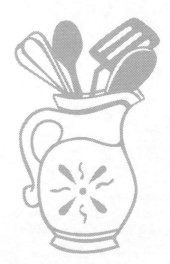

Recipe 463

Grape Baked Alaska

Place in a vitamix

1 cup of sucanant sugar
1 cup of maple syrup
1 cup of almond butter
One cup of grapes (any color)
1 Brick or one pound of Tofu

Mix and place into baking dishes 4 dishes needed
I use the same dishes for pot pies 7 x 7 inches
Bake 350 degrees 20 minutes
Let Cool serve cold or semi frozen
Freeze extra covered

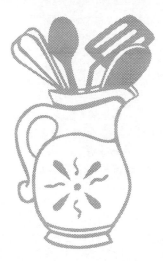

Recipe 464

Cheese Sauce for Baked Potato

Place in Microwave oven for 5 minutes the following mix:

Mix in bowl:
1 teaspoon of Biosalt
2/3 cups of cornmeal
2 cups of water

Then place in vitamix with the following:

3 tablespoons of lemon juice
1 cup of tofu
1 cup of tomatoes
¼ cup of sesame seeds
1 teaspoon of onion powder
½ teaspoon of Biosalt
½ teaspoon of garlic powder

Add 1 teaspoon at a time of water to make mixture thin
Blend until smooth

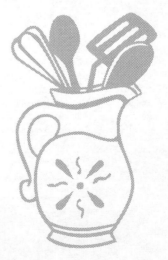

Recipe 465

Apple Ice Cream

Directions:
Place in a vitamix or blender the following:

Ingredients:
One fourth teaspoon of Biosalt
Two cups of Walnuts
One brick or one pound of Tofu
One half cup of Soy Milk
One large Apple (remove core only)
One tablespoon of Almond Butter
Two cups of Maple Syrup
Three cups of Puffed Rice

Blend until smooth and freeze.
Place in 6-ounce cups and store extra in freezer.

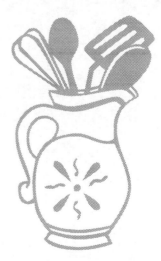

Plum Ice Cream

Directions:
Place in a vitamix or blender the following:

Ingredients:
One fourth teaspoon of Biosalt
Two cups of Walnuts
One brick or one pound of Tofu
One half cup of Soy Milk
Four plums (remove stem/seed only)
One tablespoon of Almond Butter
Two cups of Maple Syrup
Three cups of Puffed Rice

Blend until smooth and freeze.
Place in 6-ounce cups and store extra in freezer.

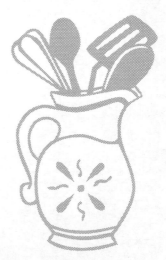

Recipe 467

Grape Ice Cream

Directions:
Place in a vitamix or blender the following:

Ingredients:
One fourth teaspoon of Biosalt
Two cups of Walnuts
One brick or one pound of Tofu
One half cup of Soy Milk
Two cups of seedless grapes
One tablespoon of Almond Butter
Two cups of Maple Syrup
Three cups of Puffed Rice

Blend until smooth and freeze. Place in 6-ounce cups and store extra in freezer.

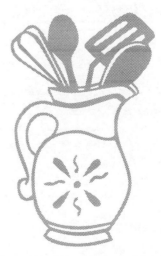

Recipe 468

Pear Ice Cream

Directions:
Place in a vitamix or blender the following:

Ingredients:
One fourth teaspoon of Biosalt
Two cups of Walnuts
One brick or one pound of Tofu
One half cup of Soy Milk
Two large pears (remove stem/seed only)
One tablespoon of Almond Butter
Two cups of Maple Syrup
Three cups of Puffed Rice

Blend until smooth and freeze. Place in 6-ounce cups and store extra in freezer.

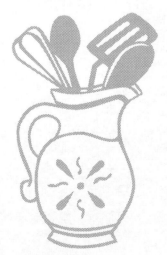

Recipe 469

R H I Maple Syrup Cookies

Mix in a large bowl the following:

1 teaspoon of vanilla
1 teaspoon of pineapple juice
1 teaspoon of biosalt
4 cups of maple syrup
4 cups of sifted whole wheat pastry flour

Mix and form cookies on trays. lined with cookie mat.

Helpful hints:
Mix dough the night before.
Place in refrigerator covered.
Bake 325 degree 25 minutes

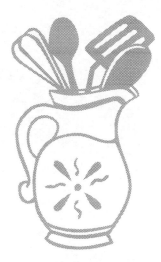

Recipe 470

Maple Syrup Brownies

Mix in a large bowl the following:

2 tablespoons of almond butter
2 tablespoons of Lemon Juice
1 teaspoon of vanilla
1 tablespoon of of biosalt
6 cups of walnuts grounded
6 cups of maple syrup
4 cups of sifted whole wheat pastry flour

Mix and pour into a glass dish 9 x 13 inches lined with parchment paper.
Bake 350 degrees 50 minutes
Use toothpick test to see if center is baked.
Let cool and cut into brownie shapes.

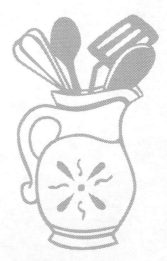

Recipe 471

Carob Nugget Candy

Place in a large bowl the following:

One half cup of carob powder
6 cups of Maple Syrup
8 tablespoons of wheat germ
2 teaspoons of Biosalt
2 teaspoons of vanilla
4 teaspoons of flaxseed meal
2 cups of walnuts chopped

Mix well and add:

4 cups of whole wheat pastry flour sifted
4 cups of oatmeal flour

Mix and pour into a glass dish 9 x 13 inches lined with parchment paper.
Bake 200 degrees for 2 and a half hours.
Let cool and place in refrigerator 24 hours.
The next day, cut into squares.

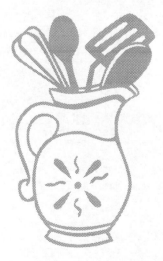

Recipe 472

Roma Nugget Candy

Place in a large bowl the following:

One half cup of Roma powder
6 cups of Maple Syrup
8 tablespoons of wheat germ
2 teaspoons of Biosalt
2 teaspoons of vanilla
4 teaspoons of flaxseed meal
2 cups of walnuts chopped

Mix well and add:

4 cups of whole wheat pastry flour sifted
4 cups of oatmeal flour

Mix and pour into a glass dish 9 x 13 inches lined with parchment paper.
Bake 200 degrees for 2 and a half hours
Let cool and place in refrigerator 24 hours.
The next day cut into squares.

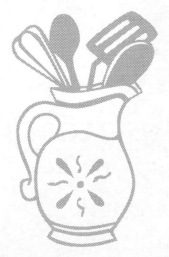

Recipe 473

Peppermint Nugget Candy

Place in a large bowl the following:

One fourth to One half teaspoon of Peppermint Oil
(On first recipe use one fourth teaspoon and on second recipe add more if desired)
6 cups of Maple Syrup
8 tablespoons of wheat germ
2 teaspoons of Biosalt
2 teaspoons of vanilla
4 teaspoons of flaxseed meal
2 cups of walnuts chopped

Mix well and add:

4 cups of whole wheat pastry flour sifted
4 cups of oatmeal flour

Mix and pour into a glass dish 9 x 13 inches lined with parchment paper.
Bake 200 degrees 2 and a half hours
Let cool and place in refrigerator 24 hours.
The next day cut into squares.

Cinnamon Nugget Candy

Place in a large bowl the following:

3 tablespoons of cinnamon
6 cups of Maple Syrup
8 tablespoons of wheat germ
2 teaspoons of Biosalt
2 teaspoons of vanilla
4 teaspoons of flaxseed meal
2 cups of walnuts chopped

Mix well and add:

4 cups of whole wheat pastry flour sifted
4 cups of oatmeal flour

Mix and pour into a glass dish 9 x 13 inches lined with parchment paper.
Bake 200 degrees 2 and a half hours
Let cool and place in refrigerator 24 hours.
The next day cut into squares.

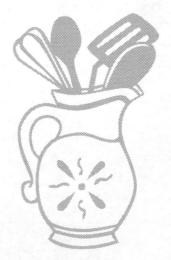

Recipe 475

Lemon Nugget Candy

Mix in a large bowl the following:

One half cup of Lemon rind
One fourth cup of Lemon Juice

6 cups of Maple Syrup
8 tablespoons of wheat germ
2 teaspoons of Biosalt
2 teaspoons of vanilla
4 teaspoons of flaxseed meal
2 cups of chopped and roasted almonds

Mix and add:

4 cups of whole wheat pastry flour sifted
4 cups of oatmeal flour

Mix and pour into a glass dish 9 x 13 inches lined with parchment paper.
Bake 200 degrees 3 hours
Let cool and place in refrigerator 24 hours.
The next day cut into squares.

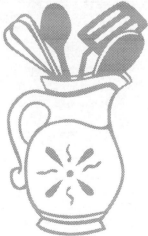

Recipe 476

Vanilla Nugget Candy

Mix in a large bowl the following:

6 cups of Maple Syrup
8 tablespoons of wheat germ
2 teaspoons of Biosalt
3 teaspoons of vanilla
4 teaspoons of flaxseed meal
2 cups of chopped and roasted almonds

Mix and add:

4 cups of whole wheat pastry flour sifted
4 cups of oatmeal flour

Mix and pour into a glass dish 9 x 13 inches lined with parchment paper.
Bake 200 degrees 2 and a half hours
Let cool and place in refrigerator 24 hours.
The next day cut into squares.

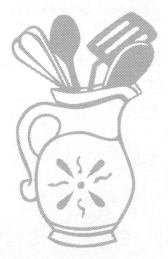

Recipe 477

Apricot Nugget Candy

Place in a large bowl the following:

6 cups of Maple Syrup
8 tablespoons of wheat germ
2 teaspoons of vanilla
4 teaspoons of flaxseed meal
2 cups of chopped walnuts

Mix and add: 6 cups of dried Apricots cut small

4 cups of whole wheat pastry flour sifted
4 cups of oatmeal flour

Mix and pour into a glass dish 9 x 13 inches lined with parchment paper.
Bake 200 degrees 2 and a half hours
Let cool and place in refrigerator 24 hours.

Italian Dry Roasted Nut Mix

In a large bowl place the following:

4 cups of each:
Almonds, walnuts, pecans.
Spray with Braggs Ammino until all nuts are covered.

The add 1 tablespoon of Biosalt.

Spray again and mix and add :
4 tablespoons of Italian Seasoning

Mix and spray again.
The add 4 cups of puffed rice.
Spray again and mix.
Place on tray lined with cookie mat
Bake 200 degrees for 12 hours or more overnight or until baked.

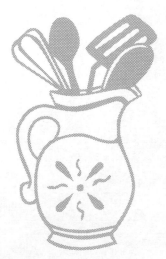

Recipe 479

Garlic Dry Roasted Puffed Corn Mix

In a large bowl pour
one bad or 6ounces of corn puffs (organic)
Spray and mix with Braggs
until all corn puffs are coated
Add one half to 1 tablespoon of garlic powder
depending on desired taste.

Mix and coat with Braggs
Add 1 teaspoon of Biosalt
Mix and spray with Braggs
Place on tray lined with cookie mat
Bake 200 degrees for 2 hours or until dry.
Let cool store in refrigerator—plastic bag

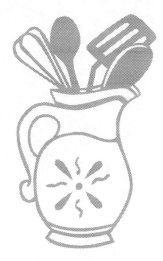

Onion Dry Roasted Puffed Corn Mix

In a large bowl pour
one bad or 6ounces of corn puffs (organic)
Spray and mix with Braggs
until all corn puffs are coated
Add one half to 1 tablespoon of onion powder
depending on desired taste.

Mix and coat with Braggs
Add 1 teaspoon of Biosalt
Mix and spray with Braggs
Place on tray lined with cookie mat
Bake 200 degrees for 2 hours or until dry.
Let cool store in refrigerator—plastic bag

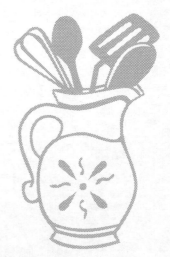

Recipe 481

Havenero Dry Roasted Puffed Corn Mix

Place into vitamix the following
one third cup of maple syrup
one third cup of lemon juice
6-12 havenero peppers

pour into a large bowl with one bag or 6 ounces of corn puffs (organic)
Spray all corn puffs with Braggs and mix.
and add:

1 teaspoon of chili powder
1 teaspoon of biosalt
1 teaspoon of onion powder
1 teaspoon of garlic powder
1 teaspoon of paprika powder
mix and spray with Braggs

Then place on a tray lined with cookie mat
Bake 200 degrees for 2 hours or until dry.
Let cool store in refrigerator—plastic bag

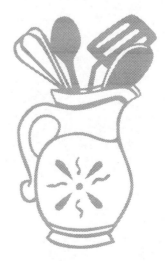

Cayenne Dry Roasted Puffed Corn Mix

Place In a large bowl pour
one bag or 6ounces of corn puffs (organic)
Spray with Braggs and mix.

Add one to 2 tablespoon of Cayenne powder

1 teaspoon of Biosalt
Mix and spray with Braggs
Pour on trays lined with cookie mat
Bake 200 degrees for 2 hours or until dry.
Let cool store in refrigerator—plastic bag

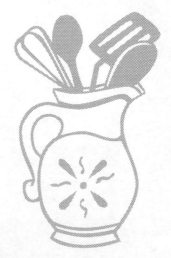

Recipe 483

Italian Dry Roasted Puffed Corn Mix

Place In a large bowl
one bag or 6 ounces of corn puffs (organic)
Spray with Braggs and mix.

Add one to 2 tablespoons of Italian seasoning

add 1 teaspoon of Biosalt
Mix and spray with Braggs
Pour on a tray lined with cookie mat
Bake 200 degrees for 2 hours or until dry.
Let cool store in refrigerator—plastic bag

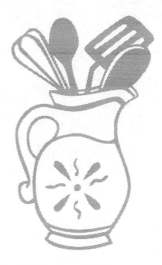

Salted Dry Roasted Puffed Corn Mix

Place In a large bowl
one bag or 6 ounces of corn puffs (organic)
Spray with Braggs and mix.

add 1 teaspoon of Biosalt
spray with Braggs and mix
Pour on a tray lined with cookie mat
Bake 200 degrees for 2 hours or until dry.
Let cool store in refrigerator—plastic bag

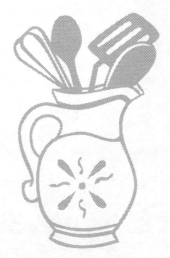

Recipe 485

Cajun Dry Roasted Puffed Corn Mix

Place In a large bowl
one bag or 6 ounces of corn puffs (organic)
Spray with Braggs and mix.

and add 1 tablespoon of the following:
garlic powder
paprika powder
onion powder
chili powder
add one teaspoon of biosalt

spray again with Braggs and mix
Pour on a tray lined with cookie mat
Bake 200 degrees for 2 hours or until dry.
Let cool store in refrigerator—plastic bag

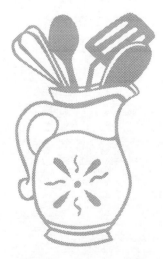

Recipe 486

Salted Havenero Dry Roasted Puffed Corn Mix

Place In a large bowl
pour one bag or 6 ounces of corn puffs (organic)
Spray with Braggs and mix.
Set aside.
Place into a vitamix the following:

6 havenero peppers
one third cup of maple syrup
one third cup of lemon juice
one teaspoon of biosalt
Mix and add to the above bowl.
Mix all ingredients and

spray again with Braggs.
Pour on a tray lined with cookie mat
Bake 200 degrees for 2 hours or until dry.
Let cool store in refrigerator—plastic bag

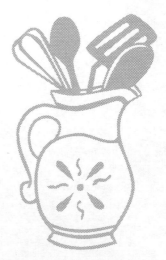

Recipe 487

Plum Tofu Cookies

(For dough see Butter Cookie Recipe #45)

Mix the night before, wrap and place iin refrigerator. The next day place 3 cups of sucanant sugar into a vitamix and make in to a fine powder.

Pour intoa large bowl and set aside.

Place one brick or one pound of Tofu and 2 cups of Plums (minus pits) into vitamix.

Blend until smooth. Place into same large bowl with sucanant sugar and add 2 cups of chopped walnuts.

MIx and set aside. If mixture is too thin add whole wheat pastry flour one tablespoon at a time.

roll out dough and with a 3 x 3 inch round cookie cutter.

cut circle in dough. Place enough mixture into center of circle and fold over.

This will look like a half moon. Press sides together and place on trays lined with cookie mat.

Bake 350 degrees 20 minutes Let cool and store in refrigerator.

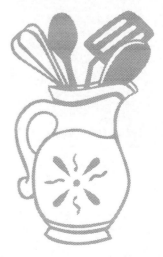

Peach Tofu Cookies

(For dough see Butter Cookie Recipe #45)

Mix the night before, wrap and place iin refrigerator. The next day place 3 cups of sucanant sugar into a vitamix and make in to a fine powder.

Pour intoa large bowl and set aside.

Place one brick or one pound of Tofu and 2 cups of Peaches (remove pits) into vitamix.

Blend until smooth. Place into same large bowl with sucanant sugar and add 2 cups of chopped walnuts.

Mix and set aside. If mixture is too thin add whole wheat pastry flour one tablespoon at a time.

roll out dough and with a 3 x 3 inch round cookie cutter.

cut circle in dough. Place enough mixture into center of circle and fold over.

This will look like a half moon. Press sides together and place on trays lined with cookie mat.

Bake 350 degrees 20 minutes Let cool and store in refrigerator.

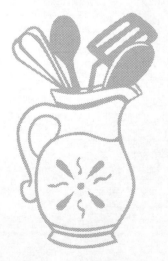

Recipe 489

Nectarine Tofu Cookies

(For dough see Butter Cookie Recipe #45)

Mix the night before, wrap and place iin refrigerator. The next day place 3 cups of sucanant sugar into a vitamix and make in to a fine powder.

Pour intoa large bowl and set aside.

Place one brick or one pound of Tofu and 2 cups of Nectarines (remove pits) into vitamix.

Blend until smooth. Place into same large bowl with sucanant sugar and add 2 cups of chopped walnuts.

MIx and set aside. If mixture is too thin add whole wheat pastry flour one tablespoon at a time.

roll out dough and with a 3 x 3 inch round cookie cutter.

cut circle in dough. Place enough mixture into center of circle and fold over.

This will look like a half moon. Press sides together and place on trays lined with cookie mat.

Bake 350 degrees 20 minutes Let cool and store in refrigerator.

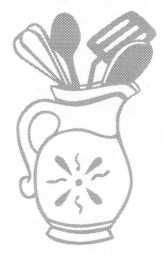

Recipe 490

Spicy Avocado Dip

Directions:

In a large bowl:

Mash four ripe avocados & add

Two jalapeno peppers cut into small pieces
Two tomato cut into small chucks
½ onion chopped
1 tablespoon of garlic powder
1 tablespoon of oregano
1 tablespoon of Braggs
4 tablespoons of lemon juice
1 teaspoon of Biosalt
1 teaspoon of dill

Mix and pour into a dish/bowl and add baked chips or see Recipe 71 for wheat chips
Cut into bite size

Helpful Hints:
Remove seeds and skin, save seeds for serving dish to keep avocado from darkening

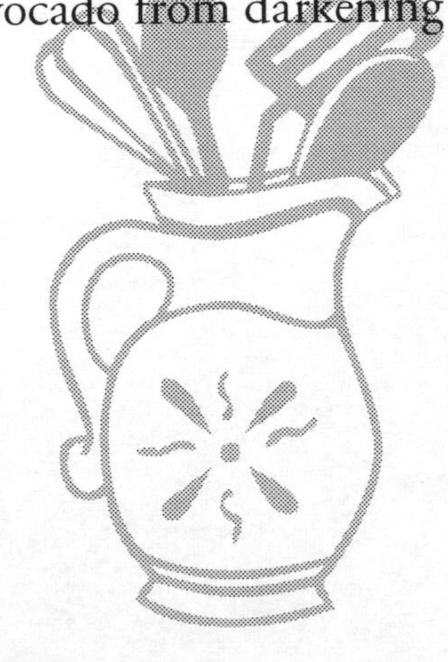

Recipe 491

All Purpose Gravy

Place the following into vitamix

1 teaspoon of garlic powder
1 teaspoon of sage
4 tablespoon of braggs
one half teaspoon of biosalt or inland sea water
one half teaspoon of thyme
one half teaspoon of Basil
2 cups of water
one half onion
1 stalk of celery
8 tablespoons of whole wheat pastry flour

Mix and pour into small pan, boil on low for 6 to 10 minutes or until thick.

Serve hot or cold.

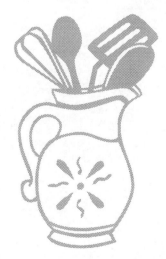

Potato and Cabbage Stew

Place the following in a large pan and boil on low for 2 hours.

20 cups of water
6 Potaotes cut into half spoon size and remove skins
One half head of green cabbage cut small
3 celery sticks cut small
2 Onions cut small
2 red peppers or one large cut small
4 cloves of garlic cut small
2 carrots shredded
6 long green onions cut small
one half cup of green peas or corn
one fourth cup of Braggs
1 tablespoon of parsley
1 tablespoon of biosalt
Mix, serve hot and add Braggs and hot sauce if desired

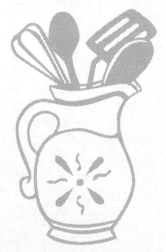

Recipe 493

Carob Pie crust

Place in a vitamix the following:

1 Tablespoon of carob powder
1 cup of oatmeal
1 cup of almonds
one fourth cup of coconut
one third teaspoon of Biosalt

Mix until the above is fine powder.
The pour into glass pie dish and add 3 tablespoons of maple syrup.
Mix and form into a pie shell
For filling see recipe # 40

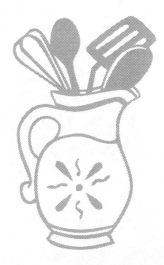

Roma Pie Crust

Place in a vitamix the following:

1 teaspoon of Roma powder
1 cup of oatmeal
1 cup of almonds
one fourth cup of coconut
one third teaspoon of Biosalt

Mix until the above until the above is a fine powder.
The pour into glass pie dish and add 3 tablespoons of maple syrup.
form into a pie shell
For filling see recipe # 495

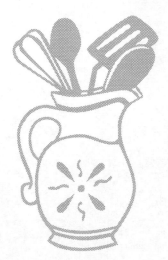

Recipe 495

Coffee Baked Pie

Place into a vitamix the following:

1 Brick or 1 pound of Tofu
1 cup of Maple Syrup
1 cup of almond butter
one half cup of Roma Coffee
one half cup of sifted whole wheat pastry flour
One half cup of sucanant sugar
For crust see Pie Crust recipe # 494

Place all the above in unbaked pie shell
Bake 350 degrees 20 minutes

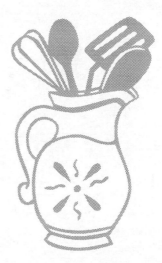

Cranberry Sauce

Place the following in a small pan. and boil for 10 minutes on low.

Stir:

4 cups or 12 ounces of fresh cranberries
1 cup of water or 1 cup of Pineapple juice

One cup of sucanant sugar
Bring to a boil and turn to low for 10-15 minutes.
Stir:
Pour into a large glass bowl.
Mash, let cool. Pour into serving bowls and place into refrigerator.

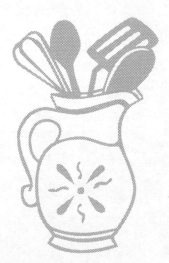

Recipe 497

Green Bean Cassrole

In a pan. boil:

1 tablespoon of Biosalt
One and half pounds of fresh cut green beans
4 cups of water

Continue to boil for 6 minutes.
Cover pan with lid. Drain water and set aside.
In a large oven bowl place the following and mix:

Three fourths cup of soymilk
three fourths cup of vegetable broth
3 cloves of garlic cut small
1 cup of olives cut each into half
1 cup of shredded carrots
2 tablespoons of whole wheat pastry flour
Mix well and add beans.
In a small bowl, mix the following:
1 and a half slices of wheat bread. Tear into small pieces.
one cup of dried onions
one eighth teaspoon of biosalt

mix and sprinkle on top,
Bake 425 degrees for 15 minutes

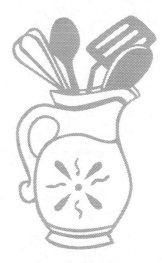

Quick Oatmeal

Place in a large bowl the following and mix:

2 cups of oatmeal
2 cups of water and 2 cups of pineapple juice
one half teaspoon of vanilla
one half teaspoon of biosalt
one half—1 teaspoon of cinnamon
one half—1 teaspoon of maple syrup

Mix and place into microwave oven for 8-10 minutes
Serve hot.

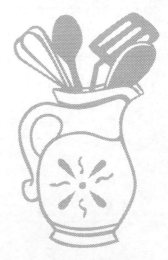

Recipe 499

Baked Yams

Cut 5-7 yams in half, place inside a glass baking dish 9 x 9 inches with lid. (can stack)
Bake 35-45 minutes 475 degrees
Remove from oven, let sit until cool,
place in refrigerator.
After baked pour one to two tablespoons of Pineappple juice on each yam.

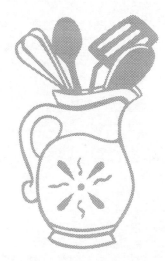

Saute Corn

IN a small pan cook corn on low for 5-10 minutes.

1 pound of corn (can be frozen)
1-2 tablespons of Braggs
4-6 tablespoons of Lemon juice
Stir and serve hot.
Can freeze extra.

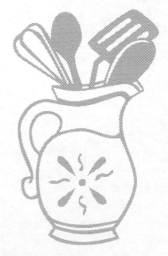

Recipe 501

Cinnamon and Ginger Cookies

Place the following in a vitamix:

1 cup of tofu
2 cups of maple syrup
4 tablespoons of soy milk
3 cups of almond butter
Blend until smooth, pour into large bowl with:
4 cups of sucanant sugar
8 teaspoons of ginger
1 teaspoon of biosalt
2 teaspoons of clove powder
4 teaspoons of cinnamon

Mix and add:
9 cups of whole wheat pastry flour sifted
Make this dough the same day of use—not the night before.
This is a dry dough. Roll dough with rolling pin, use any cookie cutter shape
    or size.
Place on cookie trays lined with cookie mat
Bake 350 degrees 8-10 minutes
Let cool for 5-10 minutes before removing from trays.

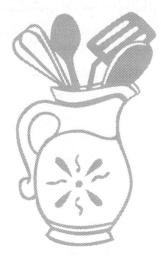

Recipe 502

Orange nugget Candy

Mix in a large bowl the following:

one half cup of Orange rind
one fourth cup of orange juice
6 cups of Maple syrup
2 teaspoons of vanilla
8 teaspoons of wheat germ
2 teaspoons of biosalt
4 teaspoons of flaxseed meal
2 cups of chopped walnuts

Mix and add:

4 cups of oatmeal flour
4 cups of whole wheat pastry flour sifted
Mix and pour into 9 x 13 inch glass dish
lined with parchment paper.

Bake 200 degrees 3 hours
Let cool
Place in refrigerator covered for 24 hours
Next day cut into squares.

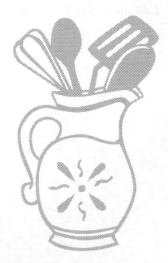

Recipe 503

Potato and Celery soup

Place following into a large pan and boil on low for one and a half to two hours.
12 cups of water
4 cups celery (chopped)
1 cup of chopped onions
6 cooked potatoes cut into bite size, remove skin
2 cloves of garlic cut small
2 tablespoons of braggs
2 tablespoons of almond butter
one tablespoon of Biosalt
2 teaspoons of hot sauce

Serve soup hot
add hot sauce and braggs if desired.
Let cool and freeze extra.

Helpful Hints: The day before place potatoes into a brown bag and microwave 8-9
    minutes or unitl cooked.
Let cool and refrigerate.

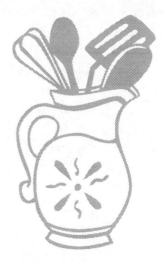

Recipe 504

Avocado Dip

Directions:

In a large bowl:

Mash four ripe avocados & add

Two tomato cut into small chucks
½ onion chopped
1 tablespoon of garlic powder
1 tablespoon of oregano
1 tablespoon of Braggs
4 tablespoons of lemon juice
1 teaspoon of Biosalt
1 teaspoon of dill

Mix and pour into a dish/bowl and add baked chips or see Recipe 71 for
     wheat chips
Cut into bite size

Helpful Hints:
Remove seeds and skin, save seeds for serving dish to keep avocado from darkening

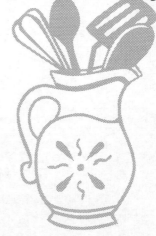

Recipe 505

Carrot soup

Place following into a large pan and boil on low for one and a half to two hours.
12 cups of water
6 carrots shredded
1 cup of chopped ionions
2 cooked potatoes cut into bite size
2 cloves of garlic cut small
2 tablespoons of braggs
4 tabelspoons of almond butter
one and a half teaspoons of biosalt
1 teaspoon of thyme
1 teaspoon of basil
1 teaspoon of marjoram
Serve soup hot
add hot sauce and braggs if desired.
Let cool and freeze extra.

Helpful Hints: The day before place potaotes into a brown bag and microwave 8-9
    minutes or unitl cooked.
Let cool and refrigerate.

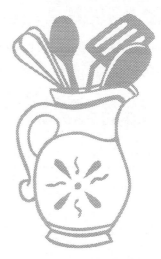

Peach Upside down Cream Cake

Mix dough first.
Place following in a vitamix:
2 cups of almond butter
12 tablespoons of pineapple juice
2 cups of maple syrup
Mix well and pour into a large bowl with:
6 cups of whole wheat pastry flour sifted
Mix and add:
Yeast (follow yeast instructions on package) or place 2 tablespoons of yeast into one half cup of finger warm water and mix.

Mix into the above bowl, cover bowl and place into a warm place.
Dough should rise in 30 minutes.

Topping: Line a round pan 10 x 10 inches with parchment paper and pour 2 cups of sucanant sugar spread even and place into vitamix: one and a half pounds of peaches (minus pits) and 1 cup of Maple syrup. Blend until smooth.
Pour into pan. Pour dough into pan. Spread evenly.

Bake 350 degrees 45-60 minutes or until baked.
Use toothpick test. Let cool for 30 minutes.
Place a large plate on top of pan then turn over.

Helpful Hints:

Turn oven lower to prevent a boil over / spill or can use a deeper pan

Recipe 507

Apricot Upside down Cream Cake

Mix dough first.
Place following in a vitamix:
2 cups of almond butter
12 tablespoons of pineapple juice
2 cups of maple syrup
Mix well and pour into a large bowl with:
6 cups of whole wheat pastry flour sifted
Mix and add:
Yeast (follow yeast instructions on package) or place 2 tablespoons of yeast into one half cup of finger warm water and mix.

Mix into the above bowl, cover bowl and place into a warm place.
Dough should rise in 30 minutes.

Topping: Line a round pan 10 x 10 inches with parchment paper and pour 2 cups of sucanant sugar spread even and place into vitamix: one and a half pounds of apricots (minus pits) and 1 cup of Maple syrup. Blend until smooth.
Pour into pan. Pour dough into pan. Spread evenly.

Bake 350 degrees 45-60 minutes or until baked.
Use toothpick test. Let cool for 30 minutes.
Place a large plate on top of pan then turn over.

Helpful Hints:

Turn oven lower to prevent a boil over / spill or can use a deeper pan

Recipe 508

Nectarine Upside down Cream Cake

Mix dough first.
Place following in a vitamix:
2 cups of almond butter
12 tablespoons of pineapple juice
2 cups of maple syrup
Mix well and pour into a large bowl with:
6 cups of whole wheat pastry flour sifted
Mix and add:
Yeast (follow yeast instructions on package) or place 2 tablespoons of yeast into one
half cup of finger warm water and mix.

Mix into the above bowl, cover bowl and place into a warm place.
Dough should rise in 30 minutes.

Topping: Line a round pan 10 x 10 inches with parchment paper and pour 2 cups
    of sucanant sugar spread even and place into vitamix: one and a half pounds of
    nectarine (minus pits) and 1 cup of Maple syrup. Blend until smooth.
Pour into pan. Pour dough into pan. Spread evenly.

Bake 350 degrees 45-60 minutes or until baked.
Use toothpick test. Let cool for 30 minutes.
Place a large plate on top of pan then turn over.

Helpful Hints:

Turn oven lower to prevent a boil over / spill or can use a deeper pan

Recipe 509

Cherry Upside down Cream Cake

Mix dough first.
Place following in a vitamix:
2 cups of almond butter
12 tablespoons of pineapple juice
2 cups of maple syrup
Mix well and pour into a large bowl with:
6 cups of whole wheat pastry flour sifted
Mix and add:
Yeast (follow yeast instructions on package) or place 2 tablespoons of yeast into one half cup of finger warm water and mix.

Mix into the above bowl, cover bowl and place into a warm place.
Dough should rise in 30 minutes.

Topping: Line a round pan 10 x 10 inches with parchment paper and pour 2 cups of sucanant sugar spread even and place into vitamix: one and a half pounds of cherry (minus pits) and 1 cup of Maple syrup. Blend until smooth.
Pour into pan. Pour dough into pan. Spread evenly.

Bake 350 degrees 45-60 minutes or until baked.
Use toothpick test. Let cool for 30 minutes.
Place a large plate on top of pan then turn over.

Helpful Hints:

Turn oven lower to prevent a boil over / spill or can use a deeper pan

Recipe 510

Grape Upside down Cream Cake

Mix dough first.

Place following in a vitamix:

2 cups of almond butter

12 tablespoons of pineapple juice

2 cups of maple syrup

Mix well and pour into a large bowl with:

6 cups of whole wheat pastry flour sifted

Mix and add:

Yeast (follow yeast instructions on package) or place 2 tablespoons of yeast into one half cup of finger warm water and mix.

Mix into the above bowl, cover bowl and place into a warm place.

Dough should rise in 30 minutes.

Topping: Line a round pan 10 x 10 inches with parchment paper and pour 2 cups of sucanant sugar spread even and place into vitamix one and a half pounds of Grapes (seedless any color) and 1 cup of Maple syrup. Blend until smooth.

Pour into pan. Pour dough into pan. Spread evenly.

Bake 350 degrees 45-60 minutes or until baked.

Use toothpick test. Let cool for 30 minutes.

Place a large plate on top of pan then turn over.

Helpful Hints:

Turn oven lower to prevent a boil over / spill or can use a deeper pan

Recipe 511

Apple Upside down Cream Cake

Mix dough first.
Place following in a vitamix:
2 cups of almond butter
12 tablespoons of pineapple juice
2 cups of maple syrup
Mix well and pour into a large bowl with:
6 cups of whole wheat pastry flour sifted
Mix and add:
Yeast (follow yeast instructions on package) or place 2 tablespoons of yeast into one half cup of finger warm water and mix.

Mix into the above bowl, cover bowl and place into a warm place.
Dough should rise in 30 minutes.

Topping: Line a round pan 10 x 10 inches with parchment paper and pour 2 cups of sucanant sugar spread even and place into vitamix: one and one half pounds of apples (minus core) and 1 cup of Maple syrup. Blend until smooth.
Pour into pan. Pour dough into pan. Spread evenly.

Bake 350 degrees 45-60 minutes or until baked.
Use toothpick test. Let cool for 30 minutes.
Place a large plate on top of pan then turn over.

Helpful Hints:

Turn oven lower to prevent a boil over / spill or can use a deeper pan

Recipe 512

Cinnamon Upside down Cream Cake

Mix dough first.
Place following in a vitamix:
2 cups of almond butter
12 tablespoons of pineapple juice
2 cups of maple syrup
Mix well and pour into a large bowl with:
6 cups of whole wheat pastry flour sifted
Mix and add:
Yeast (follow yeast instructions on package) or place 2 tablespoons of yeast into one
half cup of finger warm water and mix.

Mix into the above bowl, cover bowl and place into a warm place.
Dough should rise in 30 minutes.

Topping: Line a round pan 10 x 10 inches with parchment paper and pour 2 cups
    of sucanant sugar spread even and place into vitamix one to two tablespoons of
    Cinnamon and 1 cup of Maple syrup. Blend until smooth.
Pour into pan. Pour dough into pan. Spread evenly.

Bake 350 degrees 45-60 minutes or until baked.
Use toothpick test. Let cool for 30 minutes.
Place a large plate on top of pan then turn over.

Helpful Hints:

Turn oven lower to prevent a boil over / spill or can use a deeper pan

Recipe 513

Carob Upside down Cake

Mix dough first.
Place following in a vitamix:
2 cups of almond butter
12 tablespoons of pineapple juice
2 cups of maple syrup
Mix well and pour into a large bowl with:
6 cups of whole wheat pastry flour sifted
Mix and add:
Yeast (follow yeast instructions on package) or place 2 tablespoons of yeast into one half cup of finger warm water and mix.

Mix into the above bowl, cover bowl and place into a warm place.
Dough should rise in 30 minutes.

Topping: Line a round pan 10 x 10 inches with parchment paper and pour 2 cups of sucanant sugar spread even and place into vitamix: two to three tablespoons of carob and 1 cup of Maple syrup. Blend until smooth.
Pour into pan. Pour dough into pan. Spread evenly.

Bake 350 degrees 45-60 minutes or until baked.
Use toothpick test. Let cool for 30 minutes.
Place a large plate on top of pan then turn over.

Helpful Hints:

Turn oven lower to prevent a boil over / spill or can use a deeper pan

Recipe 514

Plum Upside down cream Cake

Mix dough first.
Place following in a vitamix:
2 cups of almond butter
12 tablespoons of pineapple juice
2 cups of maple syrup
Mix well and pour into a large bowl with:
6 cups of whole wheat pastry flour sifted
Mix and add:
Yeast (follow yeast instructions on package) or place 2 tablespoons of yeast into one half cup of finger warm water and mix.

Mix into the above bowl, cover bowl and place into a warm place.
Dough should rise in 30 minutes.

Topping: Line a round pan 10 x 10 inches with parchment paper and pour 2 cups of sucanant sugar spread even and place into vitamix: one to one half pound of plums (minus pits) and 1 cup of Maple syrup. Blend until smooth.
Pour into pan. Pour dough into pan. Spread evenly.

Bake 350 degrees 45-60 minutes or until baked.
Use toothpick test. Let cool for 30 minutes.
Place a large plate on top of pan then turn over.

Helpful Hints:

Turn oven lower to prevent a boil over / spill or can use a deeper pan

Recipe 515

Roma Upside down Cream Cake

Mix dough first.
Place following in a vitamix:
2 cups of almond butter
12 tablespoons of pineapple juice
2 cups of maple syrup
Mix well and pour into a large bowl with:
6 cups of whole wheat pastry flour sifted
Mix and add:
Yeast (follow yeast instructions on package) or place 2 tablespoons of yeast into one half cup of finger warm water and mix.

Mix into the above bowl, cover bowl and place into a warm place.
Dough should rise in 30 minutes.

Topping: Line a round pan 10 x 10 inches with parchment paper and pour 2 cups of sucanant sugar spread even and place into vitamix three to four tablespoons of Roma powder and 1 cup of Maple syrup. Blend until smooth.
Pour into pan. Pour dough into pan. Spread evenly.

Bake 350 degrees 45-60 minutes or until baked.
Use toothpick test. Let cool for 30 minutes.
Place a large plate on top of pan then turn over.

Helpful Hints:

Turn oven lower to prevent a boil over / spill or can use a deeper pan

Pineapple Upside down Cream Cake

Mix dough first.
Place following in a vitamix:
2 cups of almond butter
12 tablespoons of pineapple juice
2 cups of maple syrup
Mix well and pour into a large bowl with:
6 cups of whole wheat pastry flour sifted
Mix and add:
Yeast (follow yeast instructions on package) or place 2 tablespoons of yeast into one
half cup of finger warm water and mix.

Mix into the above bowl, cover bowl and place into a warm place.
Dough should rise in 30 minutes.

Topping: Line a round pan 10 x 10 inches with parchment paper and pour 2 cups
of sucanant sugar spread even and place into vitamix one and a half pounds of
Pineapple and 1 cup of Maple syrup. Blend until smooth.
Pour into pan. Pour dough into pan. Spread evenly.

Bake 350 degrees 45-60 minutes or until baked.
Use toothpick test. Let cool for 30 minutes.
Place a large plate on top of pan then turn over.

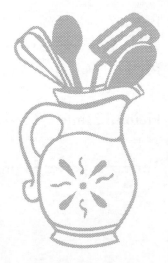

Recipe 517

Peppermint Upside down Cake

Mix dough first.
Place following in a vitamix:
2 cups of almond butter
12 tablespoons of pineapple juice
2 cups of maple syrup
Mix well and pour into a large bowl with:
6 cups of whole wheat pastry flour sifted
Mix and add:
Yeast (follow yeast instructions on package) or place 2 tablespoons of yeast into one half cup of finger warm water and mix.

Mix into the above bowl, cover bowl and place into a warm place.
Dough should rise in 30 minutes.

Topping: Line a round pan 10 x 10 inches with parchment paper and pour 2 cups
    of sucanant sugar spread even and place into vitamix: one fourth to one half
    teaspoon of liquid peppermint, and 1 cup of Maple syrup. Blend until smooth.
Pour into pan. Pour dough into pan. Spread evenly.

Bake 350 degrees 45-60 minutes or until baked.
Use toothpick test. Let cool for 30 minutes.
Place a large plate on top of pan then turn over.

Helpful Hints:

Turn oven lower to prevent a boil over / spill or can use a deeper pan

Orange Upside down Cream Cake

Mix dough first.

Place following in a vitamix:

2 cups of almond butter

12 tablespoons of pineapple juice

2 cups of maple syrup

Mix well and pour into a large bowl with:

6 cups of whole wheat pastry flour sifted

Mix and add:

Yeast (follow yeast instructions on package) or place 2 tablespoons of yeast into one half cup of finger warm water and mix.

Mix into the above bowl, cover bowl and place into a warm place.

Dough should rise in 30 minutes.

Topping: Line a round pan 10 x 10 inches with parchment paper and pour 2 cups of sucanant sugar spread even and place into vitamix one half to one cup of Orange rind and 1 cup of Maple syrup. Blend until smooth.

Pour into pan. Pour dough into pan. Spread evenly.

Bake 350 degrees 45-60 minutes or until baked.

Use toothpick test. Let cool for 30 minutes.

Place a large plate on top of pan then turn over.

Helpful Hints:

Turn oven lower to prevent a boil over / spill or can use a deeper pan

Recipe 519

Lemon Upside down Cream Cake

Mix dough first.

Place following in a vitamix:

2 cups of almond butter

12 tablespoons of pineapple juice

2 cups of maple syrup

Mix well and pour into a large bowl with:

6 cups of whole wheat pastry flour sifted

Mix and add:

Yeast (follow yeast instructions on package) or place 2 tablespoons of yeast into one half cup of finger warm water and mix.

Mix into the above bowl, cover bowl and place into a warm place.

Dough should rise in 30 minutes.

Topping: Line a round pan 10 x 10 inches with parchment paper and pour 2 cups of sucanant sugar spread even and place into vitamix one half to one cup of Lemon rind and 1 cup of Maple syrup. Blend until smooth.

Pour into pan. Pour dough into pan. Spread evenly.

Bake 350 degrees 45-60 minutes or until baked.

Use toothpick test. Let cool for 30 minutes.

Place a large plate on top of pan then turn over.

Helpful Hints:

Turn oven lower to prevent a boil over / spill or can use a deeper pan

Recipe 520

Ginger Upside down Cream Cake

Mix dough first.
Place following in a vitamix:
2 cups of almond butter
12 tablespoons of pineapple juice
2 cups of maple syrup
Mix well and pour into a large bowl with:
6 cups of whole wheat pastry flour sifted
Mix and add:
Yeast (follow yeast instructions on package) or place 2 tablespoons of yeast into one half cup of finger warm water and mix.

Mix into the above bowl, cover bowl and place into a warm place.
Dough should rise in 30 minutes.

Topping: Line a round pan 10 x 10 inches with parchment paper and pour 2 cups of sucanant sugar spread even and place into vitamix one half to one teaspoon of Ginger and 1 cup of Maple syrup. Blend until smooth.
Pour into pan. Pour dough into pan. Spread evenly.

Bake 350 degrees 45-60 minutes or until baked.
Use toothpick test. Let cool for 30 minutes.
Place a large plate on top of pan then turn over.

Helpful Hints:

Turn oven lower to prevent a boil over / spill or can use a deeper pan

Recipe 521

Jamaican Rice

The night before place 6 cups of rice and 8 cups of water into a large pan and set aside.

The next day place following into a small pan, and boil-saute for 10-15 minutes on low.

1 pound of peas—frozen ok
5 Jalapeno peppers cut small
1 onion cut small
5 long green onions cut small
One half cup of Cilantro
3 tablespoons of almond butter
3 tablespoons Braggs
1 tablespoon of Garlic powder
1 tablespoon of biosalt

Mix and set aside
Boil the rice on high, then turn to low with lid for approximately 15 minutes when cooked, pour all ingredients into pan and mix.
Turn stove off and keep lid on.
Serve hot. Can freeze extra.

Recipe 522

Lemon and Olive Basmati Rice Mix

Place into a large pan the night before the following:

6 cups of Basmanti rice
8 cups of water
1 teaspoon of biosalt

Mix and set aside.
The next day boil with lid on for 10-20 minutes or until cooked and add:

1 can of olives cut each into one half
One half cup of lemon juice

Mix and replace lid on pan and let sit for 30 minutes.

Serve hot. Can freeze extra.
(can add cilantro—one half cup cut small)

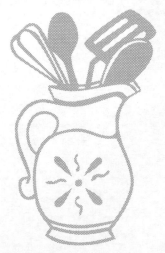

Recipe 523

Carrot and Olive Basmati Rice Mix

Place into a large pan the night before the following:

6 cups of Basmanti rice
8 cups of water
1 teaspoon of biosalt

Mix and set aside.
The next day boil on high and turn to low 10-20 minutes with lid on pan, and add:
3 carrots shredded
1 can of olives cut each into one half
Turn stove off—

Mix and place lid on pan and let sit for 30 minutes or more.

Serve hot. Can freeze extra

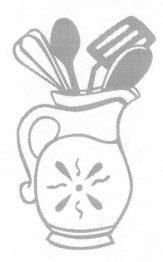

Garlic and Onion Saute Corn

IN a small pan cook corn on low for 5-10 minutes.

1 pound of corn (can be frozen)
1-2 tablespons of Braggs
4-6 tablespoons of Lemon juice
1 to 2 teaspoons garlic powder
1 to 2 teaspoons of onion powder
Stir and serve hot.
Can freeze extra.

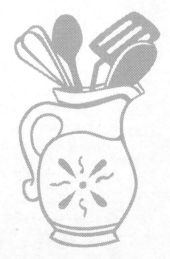

Recipe 525

Green Jalapeno Rice Mix

The night before place in a large pan the following:

6 cups of rice
8 cups of water
1 teaspoon of biosalt

Mix and set aside.
The next day place in the above pan (with lid)

1 to 2 cups of green Jalapeno peppers cut small
3 tablespoons Braggs
2 tablespoons of Oregano
1 tablespoon of Onion powder
1 tablespoon of Garlic powder

Mix and boil on high
then turn to low for 10 to 15 minutes or until rice is cooked.
Then turn heat off and let sit with lid on pan for approximately 30 minutes.
Serve hot. Can freeze extra.
Mix and set aside

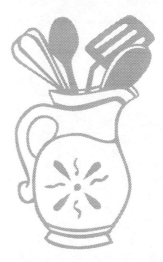

Roasted Pistachio Candy

In a large pan :

Boil for 30 minutes on warm the following:

6 cups of maple syrup

3 tablespoons of soy milk

One and a half teaspoons of Biosalt

6 tablespoons of almond butter

Stir and add 3 cups of Pistachio nuts * roasted and grounded

and boil on warm for 15 more minutes.

Add 4 teaspoons of carob powder

and boil for 15 more minutes and stir.

Add 3 cups of puffed corn and boil for 15 minutes on warm and stir.

Then turn to low and stir until thick.

Pour mixture on 2 sheets of parchment paper, lay on a counter side by side, like a sandwich.

Place 2 more sheets of parchment paper on top of mixture, and with a rolling pin roll thin.

Let cool and break into desired pieces.

Store in refrigerator

* After Pistachios are cooled place in a heavy bag and with a hammer break into smaller parts.

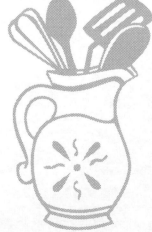

Recipe 527

Pistachio Fudge

Boil on warm for 5 minutes the following:
Two and a half cups of sucanant sugar
1 cups of maple syrup
Stir and add:
1 tablespoon of carob powder
1 tablespoon of roma powder
Boil for 5 more minutes on warm
Then add 2 cups of roasted Pistachios and boil; for 5 more minutes on warm
(after Pistachios are roasted and cooled, place into heavy bag and smash into small
    pieces)
Stir and add
Two and a half cups of almond butter and boil for 5 more minutes on warm
For a softer fudge add almond butter 5 minutes earlier.
Stir.
Pour mixture into 8 x 8 inch glass dish lined with parchment paper.
Let cool Cut into squares.

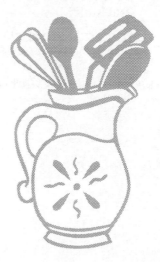

Recipe 528

Spicy Corn Bread

Place the following into vitamix

One half cup of tofu

4 cups of soymilk or water (or combination)

8 teaspoons of almond butter

2 teaspoons of sucanant sugar

4 teaspoons of biosalt

2 tablespoons of cumin

2 tablespoons of onion powder

2 tablespoons of garlic powder

2 tablespoons of chili powder

2 tablespoons of paprika

2 tablespoons of cayenne powder

2 tablespoons of Italian seasoning

Mix and pour into a large bowl and add:

2 cups of whole corn (can be frozen)

2 cups of corn meal

2 cups of whole wheat pastry flour sifted

Mix and let sit at room temperature

Then add yeast 1 tablespoon of yeast into one fourth cup of finger warm water.

Add to large bowl and let sit in warm place, covered. (or see yeast instructions on package)

Pour mixture into glass oven dish lined with parchment paper.

Bake 425 degrees 25 minutes or until baked.

DO NOT place in hot oven. Place dish in oven and turn on heat

Recipe 529

Red Hot Roast

Place the following in a large pan and boil on low for 15 minutes:

1 can of olives cut each in half

4 long green onions cut small

2 onions cut small

One half cup of cilantro cut small

3 cloves of garlic cut small

2 stalks of celery cut small

8 jalapeno peppers cut small

1 cup of peas

3 cups of walnuts chopped

2 carrots shredded

one half teaspoon of thyme

1 teaspoon of sage

1 teaspoon of marjoram

1 tablespoon of biosalt

2 tablespoons of lemon juice

2 tablespoons of braggs

2 tablespoons of cayanne pepper

1 cup of water

1 cup of pineapple juice

* stir and add Baked Rice

stir and add 1 loaf of bread

Tear each slice into 6-8 p[arts. Mix and pour all ingredients into a large oven dish
    9 x 13 inches lined with parchment paper.

With a large spoon backside press into dish.

Bake one hour at 350 degrees

* Helpful hints: The night before bake rice. Place in oven dish with lid the
    following:

4 and a half cups of water

2 cups of rice

1 teaspoon of biosalt

Bake 2 hours at 250 degrees

(if rice is gummy that is OK)

Cinnamon Walnut Cookies

Place in a large bowl the following:

2 to 4 tablespoons of cinnamon
6 cups of walnuts grounded
4 cups of maple syrup
1 teaspoon of vanilla
1 teaspoon of almond butter

Mix and add 4 cups of whole wheat pastry flour (sifted)
Mix again. Do this the day before and cover.
Place in refrigerator. The next day form on trays, 9 cookies maximum, each cookie
    one and half by one and half inches. One tray in oven at a time.
All trays lined with cookie mat.
Bake 325 degrees for 25 minutes

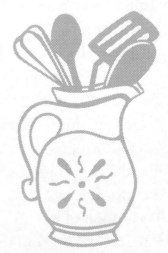

Recipe 531

Orange Ball Cookies

Mix in a large bowl the following:

3 to 5 tablespoons of orange rind
3 cups of maple syrup
3 cups of almond butter
1 cup of sucanant sugar
4 teaspoons of orange juice
2 cups of chopped walnuts
1 teaspoon of biosalt

Mix and add 4 cups of whole wheat pastry flour (sifted)
Mix again. and roll into balls. Ball size one and half by one and half inches.
Dough will be sticky, so roll in a small bowl of coconut flour.
Place on trays lined with with cookie mat.
Bake 350 degrees for 25 minutes

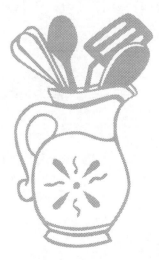

Lemon Ball Cookies

Mix in a large bowl the following:

3 to 5 tablespoons of lemon rind
3 cups of maple syrup
3 cups of almond butter
1 cup of sucanant sugar
4 teaspoons of lemon juice
2 cups of chopped walnuts
1 teaspoon of biosalt

Mix and add 4 cups of whole wheat pastry flour (sifted)
Mix again and roll into balls. Ball size: one and half by one and half inches.
Dough will be sticky, so roll in a small bowl of coconut flour.
Place on trays lined with cookie mat.
Bake 350 degrees for 25 minutes

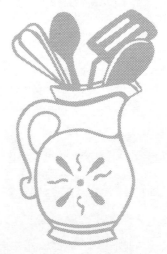

Recipe 533

Orange Pastry

CRUST:

Place in a large bowl the following:

2 cups of maple syrup
2 cups of almond butter
2 cups of walnuts grounded
2 cups of whole wheat pastry flour (sifted)

Mix and
Place on cookie tray lined with parchment paper. (tray should have 4 sides and edges)
Bake 350 degrees for 25 minutes

FOR TOPPING:

Place in a vitamix the following:

6 tablespoons of orange juice
6 tablespoons of orange rind
2 cups of maple syrup
1 cup of sucanant sugar
1 brick or 1 pound of tofu
One third cup of whole wheat pastry flour (sifted)

Mix and add topping to baked crust, add another 2 cups of chopped walnuts on top.
Return to oven at 350 degrees for 25 to 30 minutes

Recipe 534

Cinnamon Macroons

Mix the following the day before and place covered in refrigerator:

3 tablespoons of cinnamon
6 cups of maple syrup
1 teaspoon of biosalt
2 teaspoons of almond butter
4 cups of coconut

Mix and add 5 cups of whole wheat pastry flour (sifted)
Form and place on trays , 2 spoons of the mixture,
Form into a circle . . . . 9 per tray. All trays lined with a cookie mat.
Bake 325 degrees for 25 minutes

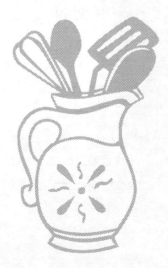

Recipe 535

Cinnamon and Oatmeal cookies

Place in a large bowl the following:

2 teaspoons of vanilla
4 tablespoons of cinnamon
6 cups of maple syrup
2 teaspoon of biosalt
8 teaspoons of almond butter
8 cups of oatmeal flour
4 cups of whole wheat pastry flour (sifted)

Mix and place in refrigerator covered. Do this the day before.
The next day form cookies on trays lined with cookie mat. 9 per tray cookie size
    one and half by one and a half inches.
Bake 325 degrees for 20 minutes

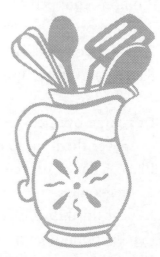

Red Potato Casserole

THE SAUCE
Place the following into vitamix until smooth :

2 teaspoons of biosalt
3 tablespoons of corn starch
2 tablespoons of paprica
2 tablespoons of chili powder
1 tablespoon of red pepper flakes
1 teaspoon of marjoram
1 teaspoon of thyme
1 teaspoon of sage
1 tespoon of garlic powder
one half cup of cleaned cashews
2 cups of water
2 cups of hot sauce

Blend and add 3 more cups of water and set aside.
Slice very thin 10 to 16 red cleaned potatoes (slice on angle) and nset aside. In a
    medium pan boil:

2 stalks of of celery chopped
2 onions chopped
2 bell peppers chopped
2 tablespoons of Braggs
Saute for 10 to 15 minutes.

In a large oven casserole glass dish 9 by 13 inches place enough of above sauce to
    cover the bottom of dish, then place slices of potatoes to cover sauce.
Place a layer of vegetables on top of potatoes and then add sauce to cover
    vegetables.
Repeat until dish is full.
(Sauce, potatoes, onions, bell peppers, celery, potato, sauce.)
Bake 350 degrees 90 minutes

Recipe 537

Cinnamon Ice cream

Place into vitamix the following:

One fourth teaspoon of biosalt
2 cups of walnuts
1 brick or 1 pound of tofu
One half cup or more soymilk
1 to 2 tablespoons of cinnamon (depending on taste)
3 cups of puffed rice
2 cups of maple syrup
1 tablespoon of almond butter

Blend until smooth
Pour into jars one half pint and freeze.

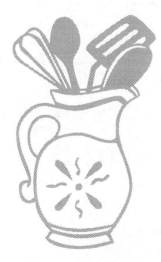

Recipe 538

Date Walnut Tart

Crust
Place in a large bowl the following and mix:

1 cup of almond butter
4 tabelspoons of maple syrup
One fourth teaspoon of biosalt
1 teaspoon of vanilla
2 cups of sifted whole wheat pastry flour

Mix and place in a 12 x 7 inch dish lined with parchment paper.
Bake 10 minutes at 350 degrees

Topping
Boil the following for 10 minutes on low.

3 cups of maple syrup
4 teaspoons of ginger
one half cup of carob
4 cups of walnuts chopped
1 cup of dates cut small (remove pitts)

Pour mixture on baked crust spread evenly.
Return to oven for 8 more minutes at 400 degrees.

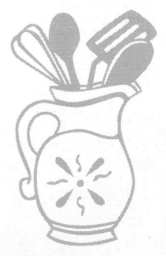

Recipe 539

Walnut Ginger Cookies

Mix the following in a large bowl:

2-4 teaspoons of ginger
1 teaspoon of vanilla
1 tablespoon of soymilk
1 tablespoon of almond butter
1 tablespoon of biosalt
6 cups of ground walnuts
4 cups of maple syrup
4 cups of whole wheat pastry flour sifted

If dough is sticky let sit for 2 hours or more. Form in cookies on trays lined with
    cookie mat 9 per tray.
Bake 325 degrees for 25 minutes

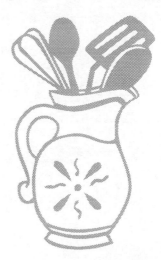

Recipe 540

Walnut Roma Cookies

Place in a large bowl the following:

6 tablespoons of roma powder
1 tablespoon of soymilk
1 tablespoon of almond butter
1 tablespoon of biosalt
1 teaspoon of vanilla
6 cups of ground walnuts
4 cups of whole wheat pastry flour sifted

If dough is sticky let sit for 2 hours or more. Form in cookies on trays lined with
    cookie mat 9 per tray.
Bake 325 degrees for 25 minutes

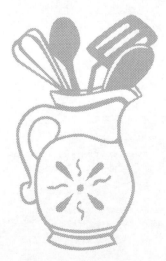

Recipe 541

Walnut Carob Cookies

Mix the following in a large bowl:

6 tablespoons of Carob powder
1 teaspoon of vanilla
1 tablespoon of soymilk
1 tablespoon of almond butter
1 tablespoon of biosalt
6 cups of ground walnuts
4 cups of maple syrup
4 cups of whole wheat pastry flour sifted

If dough is sticky let sit for 2 hours or more. Form in cookies on trays lined with cookie mat 9 per tray.
Bake 325 degrees for 25 minutes

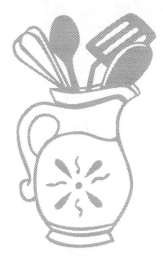

Spice Walnut Cookies

Mix the following in a large bowl:
1 teaspoon of ginger
1 teaspoon of clove powder
1 teaspoon of cinnamon
1 tablespoon of soymilk
1 tablespoon of almond butter
1 tablespoon of biosalt
1 teaspoon of vanilla
6 cups of ground walnuts
4 cups of whole wheat pastry flour sifted
6 cups of maple syrup

Mix and form cookies on trays lined with cookie mat. 9 per tray.
(if dough is too sticky let sit for 2 hours or more)
Bake 325 degrees for 25 minutes

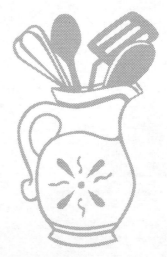

Recipe 543

Lemon and Herb Dry Roasted Nut Mix

Place the following and mix in a large bowl:

4 cups of walnuts
4 cups of pecans
4 cups of almonds
Spray with Braggs until all nuts are wet.
Mix and add:
One half cup of lemon powder
1 tablespoon of biosalt
4 tablespoons of Italian dressing

Mix and spray again with Braggs.
Mix and add:

3 cups of Puffed corn or puffed rice

Spray again with Braggs until all ingredients are wet,
Place on tray lined with cookie mat.
Bake 200 degrees 12 hours or more until crisp.

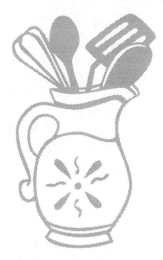

RECIPE LIST

1.   BAKED POTATO
2.   SALADS
3.   PASTA
4.   PASTA SAUCE—TOMATO SAUCE
5.   BROWN RICE
6.   TEXAN RICE
7.   BELL PEPPER RICE
8.   TOSTADAS
9.   POPCORN
10. HOT SAUCE
11. CINDY HUCK BEANS FOR BURRITOS
12. TODD NEUMILLER CHINESE SOUP
13. ALMOND BUTTER
14. PIZZA SAUCE
15. PIZZA DOUGH (FOR PIES)
16. WAFFLES
17. TAMALE CASSEROLE
18. MAPLE SYRUP CAKE
19. PAN—FRIED NOODLES
20. FRUIT ICING
21. CAROB BAKED ALASKA
22. VANILLA CAKE
23. CAROB GLAZE
24. MAPLE OATMEAL CAKE
25. CLOVE COOKIES
26. DONALD W. HUCK COCONUT COOKIES
27. CAROB ROMA OATMEAL COOKIES
28. DEEP—DISH PIZZA
29. COCONUT OATMEAL CAROB ROMA COOKIES
30. COCONUT OATMEAL COOKIES
31. CAROB ROMA COCONUT OATMEAL WHOLE-WHEAT PASTRY
     FLOUR COOKIES

32. COCONUT OATMEAL WHOLE WHEAT PASTRY FLOUR COOKIES
33. STUFFED BELL PAPPERS
34. MAPLE SYRUP COOKIES
35. CAROB COOKIES
36. CAROB BROWN CAKE
37. ANY FRUIT COOKIES (PEACH, CHERRY, APRICOT)
38. SPECIAL PIE CRUST
39. PUMPKIN PIE
40. PARVIN MALEK CAROB PIE
41. ALMOND BUTTER COOKIES 2
42. CAROB FILLING
43. EVELYN ANN MENZIE OLD-FASHIONED GLAZE
44. PINEAPPLE PIE
45. BUTTER COOKIES
46. SUCANANT COOKIES
47. INEZ A. MENZIE COCONUT COOKIES
48. TURNOVERS
49. GOLDEN MACAROONS
50. ORIENTAL CRUNCH
51. PINEAPPLE CANDY
52. CAROB DOUGHNUTS
53. LEMON DOUGHNUTS
54. GRAIN PIZZA
55. CORNMEAL PIZZA
56. CAROB BROWNIES
57. ROBERT E MENZIE WALNUT PIE
58. APRICOT COCONUT WALNUT SQUARES
59. PISTACHIO SCONES
60. EGG ROLLS
61. ROASTED SALTED NUTS
62. FUDGE CUP COOKIE
63. FUDGE SAUCE
64. PINEAPPLE COOKIES
65. TAMALE BEAN PIE
66. NUT PIE

67. DATE WALNUT COOKIES
68. CARAMELIZED GINGER HAZELNUT TART
69. PAPAYA COOKIES
70. CAJUN MIXED NUTS
71. TACO SALAD SHELLS
72. FOR CAKE-WEDDING STYLE CAKE
73. SPANISH MILLET CASSEROLE
74. ENCHILADAS
75. CAROB PIE
76. NUT BUTTER BALLS
77. SHARAREH SHABAFROOZ GARLIC BREAD SPREAD/BUTTER
78. GLAZED CARROT CAKE
79. WAFFLES WITH CASHEWS AND OATMEAL
80. LEMON PINEAPPLE PIE
81. CORN BREAD
82. MATTHEW F. MOONEY ROAST FOR ANY HOLIDAY
83. SPICE DOUGHNUTS
84. SPANISH RICE
85. PINEAPPLE SANDWICH COOKIE
86. CAROB CUP COOKIE
87. ANY FRUIT CUP COOKIE
88. SETAREH TAIS CAKE
89. CAROB DATE PISTACHIO PASTRY
90. FRUIT CAKE COOKIE
91. BAKED MILLET
92. BISCOTTI
93. MULTIGRAIN CRACKERS
94. POT PIE
95. BASIC COOKIE WITH FROSTING
96. TACO SHELLS
97. ANY FRUIT PASTRY
98. PINEAPPLE FROSTING
99. PINEAPPLE UPSIDE DOWN CAKE
100. HOT BEANS FOR BURRITOS
101. APRICOT PIE
102. APPLE PIE

103. PLUM PIE

104. PIZZA SAUCE NO. 3

105. PIZZA SAUCE NO. 1

106. COFFEE MUFFINS

107. GLORIA DUGGINS PECAN CANDY

108. PETER P. PANAGOPOULOS ALMOND FUDGE

109. PETE/ROSA CERRILLO CINNAMON WALNUT CANDY

110. SUGARED NUTS

111. PAPAYA CANDY

112. CAROB CAKE

113. THELMA MAIN HAZELNUT FUDGE

114. WHEAT CORNMEAL PIZZA

115. MARGARET/HARVEY BINDER PECAN FUDGE

116. MICHAEL F. MOONEY PECAN ROMA CAROB CANDY

117. BELLE HUCK WALNUT FUDGE

118. SAUCE FOR INSIDE CINNAMON ROLLS

119. NECTARINE PIE

120. COOKIES/CAROB PLAIN OR ROMA

121. CAROB BARS

122. SPICE BUTTER COOKIES

123. OAT CRACKERS

124. CINNAMON SUGAR DOUGHNUT TOPPING

125. JELLY DOUGHNUT FILLING

126. STRUDEL DOUGH

127. DATE CUP COOKIE

128. ITALIAN SAUCE

129. 129 LASAGNA

130. BOB PANAGOPOULOS PIZZA SAUCE NO. 2

131. CUBAN BLACK BEANS IN RICE

132. BLACK BEANS

133. LIGHT FUDGE

134. DARK FUDGE

135. PIGEON BEANS

136. XENIA PANAGOPOULOS PIGEON RICE

137. ALEXANDRA PANAGOPOULOS SWEET AND SOUR SAUCE NO. 1

138. INEZ SPEIDELL SWEET AND SOUR SAUCE NO. 2

139. VERY VERY HOT SAUCE
140. LENTILS
141. SHRIMP SAUCE
142. ALMOND CAROB CANDY
143. CAROB ROMA CANDY
144. WALNUT CINNAMON CLUSTERS
145. TAMARA NEUMILLER SPANISH PASTA
146. CHINESE RICE
147. CHILI BEANS
148. TAMALES
149. VEGETABLE SOUP
150. CAROB ROMA COOKIES
151. RAY AND LINDA PANAGOPOULOS SUNFLOWER COCONUT WAFFLES
152. WAFFLES OATMEAL AND ALMONDS
153. RHI CAROB AND ROMA OATMEAL WWP NUTLESS COOKIE
154. HOT SAUCE
155. RED BEANS FOR TOP OF RICE
156. CORN MEAL WAFFLES
157. TAGLIATELLE SAUCE
158. ALMOND BUTTER COOKIES
159. MAPLE SYRUP FROSTING
160. ORANGE GLAZE
161. RYE PANCAKES
162. PANCAKES
163. BLUEBERRY TOPPING
164. ROMA ICE CREAM
165. LEMON ICE CREAM
166. ORANGE DATE SYRUP
167. CAROB FUDGE SAUCE
168. COCONUT LIME FROSTING
169. CREAMY FROSTING
170. WHIPPED CREAM
171. COCONUT CREAM TOPPING NO. 1
172. COCONUT CREAM TOPPING NO. 2
173. MOHAMAD-TAGHI MALEK CAROB MOUSSE

209. ALMOND BUTTER FROSTING
210. CRUNCH TOPPING FOR ANY BAKED PIE
211. CHERI GILBERT COOKED CAROB GLAZE
212. SUCANANT SUGAR GLAZE
213. ROMA CREAM FROSTING
214. LEMON FILLING
215. BAR-B-QUE SAUCE
216. TOFU FROSTING
217. SWEET SUGAR ICING
218. BLACK EYED IN RICE
219. SOY MILK CORNBREAD
220. OATMEAL ALMOND COOKIE
221. SPICED CUPCAKES
222. DATE OATMEAL COOKIE
223. ORANGE COCONUT COOKIE
224. DATE COOKIE BAR
225. APRICOT COOKIE BAR
226. GINGER PANCAKES
227. LEMON PASTRY
228. LEMON SUGAR COOKIES
229. DATE BROWNIES
230. ORIGINAL SALT WATER TAFFY
231. AURA VICTORIA HUCK PEPPERMINT SALT WATER TAFFY
232. LEMON SALT WATER TAFFY
233. VANILLA SALT WATER TAFFY
234. ORANGE SALT WATER TAFFY
235. JACK PANAGOPOULOS ROMA SALT WATER TAFFY
236. ADRIANA CERRILLO PECAN SALT WATER TAFFY
237. ELMER LYLE MENZIE ALMOND SALT WATER TAFFY
238. ASHLEY SPEIDELL WALNUT SALT WATER TAFFY
239. ROSS H. MENZIE CAROB SALT WATER TAFFY
240. COCONUT SALT WATER TAFFY
241. CINAMMON SALT WATER TAFFY
242. GINGER SALT WATER TAFFY
243. GENE KOENIG ENGLISH TOFFEE CANDY
244. LUCILLE GILBERT LEMON CHEESECAKE

245. ORANGE CHEESECAKE

246. ASHER MICHAEL NEUMILLER CAROB CHEESECAKE

247. ALLIE NICOLE BLUMA NEUMILLER CAROB CAKE

248. DR. EDE VANILLA SUGAR CAKE

249. WALNUT SQUARE COOKIES

250. TARA SHABAFROOZ PECAN SQUARE COOKIES

251. ALMOND SQUARE COOKIES

252. MARGRET ANN MENZIE PECAN ROPE COOKIES

253. MASSOOD SHABAFROOZ WALNUT ROPE COOKIES

254. ALMOND ROPE COOKIES

255. RHI COCONUT OATMEAL CAROB AND ROMA COOKIES

256. RHI COCONUT OATMEAL COOKIES

257. RHI COCONUT OATMEAL WHOLE WHEAT PASTRY FLOUR COOKIES

258. RHI CAROB COCONUT COOKIES

259. RHI COCONUT COOKIES

260. RHI CAROB AND ROMA OATMEAL COOKIES

261. RHI VANILLA DONUTS OR CAKE

262. RHI CAROB BROWN CAKE

263. RHI GOLDEN MACROONS

264. RHI COFFEE MUFFINS

265. RHI SPICED CUP CAKES

266. PEPPERMINT WALNUT FUDGE

267. PEPPERMINT ICE CREAM

268. CAROB AND ROMA ICE CREAM

269. CHERRY FUDGE

270. CAROB ROMA PEPPERMINT ICE CREAM

271. PEACH APRICOT PIE

272. ROMA BAKED ALASKA

273. RAISIN BAR COOKIES

274. FREDERICK HUCK POCKET BREAD FOLDING DIAGRAM

275. NOOSHIN MALEK SEE MOUSEH

276. ZOHREH EHSANI BLUEBERRY ICE CREAM

277. POCKET PIZZA ONE

278. RAISIN CREAM PIE

279. DR. EDE KOENIG BEEROCK

280. DATE CREAM PIE
281. POCKET RAISIN PASTRY
282. POCKET PIZZA 3
283. POCKET PIZZA 4
284. POCKET PIZZA 2
285. POCKET DATE PASTRY
286. POCKET PLUM PASTRY
287. PLUM CREAM PIE
288. POCKET CAROB PASTRY
289. POCKET ROMA PASTRY
290. POCKET WALNUT PASTRY
291. POCKET APRICOT PASTRY
292. POCKET CHERRY PASTRY
293. POCKET PEACH PASTRY
294. POCKET PINEAPPLE—LEMON PASTRY
295. POCKET PUMPKIN PASTRY
296. POCKET APPLE PASTRY
297. POCKET EGG ROLLS
298. POCKET BEAN BURRITO
299. APRICOT CREAM PIE
300. VERA WALDSCHMIDT CHERRY CREAM PIE
301. PEACH CREAM PIE
302. APPLE CREAM PIE
303. TAHEREH TAHERIAN HAVANERO HOT SAUCE
304. SHAHNAZ SHAINEE HOT AND SPICY PINTO BEANS
305. PAYAM MALEK ZADEH CAROB WHEAT COOKIES
306. RAISIN ICE CREAM
307. TOMATO CASSEROLE
308. RAISIN FACE COOKIE
309. DATE FACE COOKIE
310. PINEAPPLE COCONUT SQUARES
311. ORANGE PINEAPPLE ICE CREAM
312. LEMON PINEAPPLE ICE CREAM
313. ROMA FACE COOKIE
314. CAROB FACE COOKIE
315. PUMPKIN FACE COOKIE

316. PINEAPPLE FACE COOKIE
317. APPLE FACE COOKIE
318. PEACH FACE COOKIE
319. APRICOT FACE COOKIE
320. PLUM FACE COOKIE
321. CHERRY FACE COOKIE
322. WALNUT DOME COOKIES
323. ALMOND DOME COOKIES
324. PECAN DOME COOKIES
325. CAROB DOME COOKIES
326. ROMA DOME COOKIES
327. COFFEE CUP COOKIE
328. RAISIN CUP COOKIE
329. WALNUT CUP COOKIE
330. POCKET PASTA NO. 4
331. POCKET PASTA NO. 2
332. POCKET PASTA NO. 3
333. POCKET PASTA NO. 1
334. BRAZIL NUT CARMEL CANDY
335. HAVANERO BAKED RICE
336. MACADAMA CARMEL CANDY
337. CINNAMON CARMEL CANDY
338. WALNUT CARMEL CANDY
339. COCONUT CARMEL CANDY
340. PECAN CARMEL CANDY
341. PISTACHIO CARMEL CANDY
342. HAZEL NUT CARMEL CANDY
343. CASHEW CARMEL CANDY
344. ROASTED ALMOND CARMEL CANDY
345. LEMON CARMEL CANDY
346. ORANGE CARMEL CANDY
347. CAROB CARMEL CANDY
348. ROMA CARMEL CANDY
349. PEPPERMINT CARMEL CANDY
350. GINGER CARMEL CANDY
351. HERBS & GARLIC BAKED RICE

352. WALNUT & ALMOND FROSTING
353. PINEAPPLE & LEMON GLAZE
354. ROMA TOFU COOKIES
355. CAROB TOFU COOKIES
356. CINNAMON TOFU COOKIES
357. RAISIN TOFU COOKIES
358. APRICOT TOFU COOKIES
359. DATE TOFU COOKIES
360. CRANBERRIE TOFU COOKIES
361. SPICE TOFU COOKIES
362. PAPAYA TOFU COOKIES
363. COCONUT TOFU COOKIES
364. LEMON TOFU COOKIES
365. ORANGE TOFU COOKIES
366. PINEAPPLE TOFU COOKIES
367. BLACK BEAN SOUP
368. LEMON COCONUT COOKIES
369. CHERRY SUGAR COOKIES
370. ORANGE SUGAR COOKIES
371. RAISIN SUGAR COOKIES
372. ROMA SUGAR COOKIES
373. APPLE SUGAR COOKIES
374. CAROB SUGAR COOKIES
375. PEPPERMINT SUGAR COOKIES
376. BLUEBERRY SUGAR COOKIE
377. DATE SUGAR COOKIE
378. PINEAPPLE SUGAR COOKIE
379. PLUM SUGAR COOKIE
380. PEACH SUGAR COOKIE
381. APRICOT SUGAR COOKIE
382. NECTURINE SUGAR COOKIE
383. CRANBERRY SUGAR COOKIE
384. PUMPKIN SUGAR COOKIE
385. COCONUT CAROB CARMEL CANDY
386. COCONUT LEMON CARMEL CANDY
387. COCONUT CINNAMON CARMEL CANDY

388. COCONUT ORANGE CARMEL CANDY

389. COCONUT PEPPERMINT CARMEL CANDY

390. COCONUT ROMA CARMEL CANDY

391. COCONUT GINGER CARMEL CANY

392. DATE OATMEAL COOKIE

393. RAISIN OATMEAL COOKIE

394. WALNUT DATE COOKIE

395. WALNUT LEMON COOKIE

396. WALNUT RAISIN COOKIE

397. WALNUT ORANGE COOKIE

398. WALNUT CHERRY COOKIE

399. COCONUT DATE COOKIE

400. COCONUT CHERRY COOKIE

401. COCONUT RAISIN COOKIE

402. ONION DRIED ROASTED NUTS

403. GARLIC DRIED ROASTED NUTS

404. HAVANERO DRIED ROASTED NUTS

405. CAYENNE DRIED ROASTED NUTS

406. BLACK BEAN RICE

407. SALTED-HAVANERO DRIED ROASTED NUT MIX

408. MAPLE SYRUP DRIED ROASTED NUTS

409. CAROB MACROONS

410. LEMON MACROONS

411. ROMA MACROONS

412. ORANGE MACROONS

413. PEPPERMINT FROSTING

414. PINEAPPLE-LEMON BAKED ALASKA

415. LEMON BAKED ALASKA

416. ORANGE BAKED ALASKA

417. PEPERMINT BAKED ALASKA

418. VANILLA BAKED ALASKA

419. RED HOT FIRE SAUCE

420. APRICOT ICE CREAM

421. TWICE COOKED HERB POTATO

422. PEPPERMINT MACROONS

423. PEACH ICE CREAM

424. TWICE COOKED SPICY POTATO

425. PLUM MACROONS

426. SPICY GARLIC SPREAD

427. ITALIAN SPREAD

428. WALNUT WAFFLES

429. POPPY SEED WAFFLES

430. PUMPKIN SEED WAFFLES

431. CAROB SUCANAT SUGAR COOKIE

432. ROMA SUCANAT SUGAR COOKIE

433. PEPPERMINT SUCANAT SUGAR COOKIE

434. CINNAMON SUCANAT SUGAR COOKIE

435. GINGER SUCANAT SUGAR COOKIE

436. CAROB SUGARED NUTS

437. ROMA SUGARED NUTS

438. PECAN PIE

439. BLUEBERRY CREAM PIE

440. GRAPE PIE

441. LEMON FROSTING

442. ORANGE CAKE FROSTING

443. VANILLA CAKE FROSTING

444. PEACH MAPLE CAKE

445. PLUM MAPLE CAKE

446. APRICOT MAPLE CAKE

447. PINEAPPLE MAPLE CAKE

448. APPLE MAPLE CAKE

449. CHERRY MAPLE CAKE

450. NECTARINE MAPLE CAKE

451. LEMON MAPLE CAKE

452. ORANGE MAPLE CAKE

453. BLUEBERRY MAPLE CAKE

454. PEAR MAPLE CAKE

455. BLUEBERRY BAKED ALASKA

456. BARBEQUE HOT SAUCE

457. PISTACHIO WAFFLES

458. PEACH BAKED ALASKA

459. APRICOT BAKED ALASKA

460. APPLE BAKED ALASKA

461. PLUM BAKED ALASKA

462. NECTARINE BAKED ALASKA

463. GRAPE BAKED ALASKA

464. CHEESE SAUCE FOR BAKED POTATO

465. APPLE ICE CREAM

466. PLUM ICE CREAM

467. GRAPE ICE CREAM

468. PEAR ICE CREAM

469. RHI MAPLE SYRUP COOKIES

470. MAPLE SYRUP BROWNIES

471. CAROB NUGGET CANDY

472. ROMA NUGGET CANDY

473. PEPPERMINT NUGGET CANDY

474. CINNAMON NUGGET CANDY

475. LEMON NUGGET CANDY

476. VANILLA NUGGET

477. APRICOT NUGGET CANDY

478. ITALIAN DRY ROASTED NUT MIX

479. GARLIC DRY ROASTED PUFF CORN MIX

480. ONION DRY ROASTED PUFF CORN MIX

481. HAVENERO DRY ROASTED PUFF CORN MIX

482. CAYENNE DRY ROASTED PUFF CORN MIX

483. ITALIAN DRY ROASTED PUFF CORN MIX

484. SALTED DRY ROASTED PUFF CORN MIX

485. CAJUN DRY ROASTED PUFF CORN MIX

486. SALTED HAVENERO DRY ROASTED PUFF C CORN MIX

487. PLUM TOFU COOKIES

488. PEACH TOFU COOKIES

489. NECTARINE TOFU COOKIES

490. SPICY AVOCADO DIP

491. ALL-PURPOSE GRAVY

492. POTATO AND CABBAGE STEW

493. CAROB PIE CRUST

494. ROMA PIE CRUST

495. COFFEE BAKED PIE

496. CRANBERRY SAUCE

497. GREEN BEANS CASSEROLE

498. QUICK OATMEAL

499. BAKED YAMS

500. SAUTÉ CORN

501. CINNAMON AND GINGER COOKIES

502. ORANGE NUGGET CANDY

503. POTATO AND CELERY SOUP

504. AVOCADO DIP

505. CARROT SOUP

506. PEACH UPSIDE DOWN CREAM CAKE

507. APRICOT UPSIDE DOWN CREAM CAKE

508. NECTARINE UPSIDE DOWN CREAM CAKE

509. CHERRY UPSIDE DOWN CREAM CAKE

510. GRAPE UPSIDE DOWN CREAM CAKE

511. APPLE UPSIDE DOWN CREAM CAKE

512. CINNAMON UPSIDE DOWN CREAM CAKE

513. CAROB UPSIDE DOWN CREAM CAKE

514. PLUM UPSIDE DOWN CREAM CAKE

515. ROMA UPSIDE DOWN CREAM CAKE

516. PINEAPPLE UPSIDE DOWN CREAM CAKE

517. PEPPERMINT UPSIDE DOWN CREAM CAKE

518. ORANGE UPSIDE DOWN CREAM CAKE

519. LEMON UPSIDE DOWN CREAM CAKE

520. GINGER UPSIDE DOWN CREAM CAKE

521. JAMAICAN RICE

522. LEMON AND OLIVE BASMATI RICE MIX

523. CARROT AND OLIVE BASMATI RICE MIX

524. GARLIC AND ONION SAUTÉED CORN

525. GREEN JALAPENO RICE MIX

526. ROASTED PISTACHIO CANDY

527. PISTACHIO FUDGE

528. SPICY CORN BREAD

529. RED HOT ROAST

530. CINNAMON WALNUT COOKIES

531. ORANGE BALL COOKIES

532. LEMON BALL COOKIES

533. ORANGE PASTRY

534. CINNAMON MACROONS

535. CINNAMON AND OATMEAL COOKIES

536. RED POTATO CASSEROLE

537. CINNAMON ICE CREAM

538. DATE WALNUT TART

539. WALNUT GINGER COOKIES

540. WALNUT ROMA COOKIES

541. WALNUT CAROB COOKIES

542. SPICE WALNUT COOKIES

543. LEMON AND HERB DRY ROASTED NUT MIX

544. LEMON AND DILL DRY ROASTED NUT MIX

545. LEMON AND SALTED DRY ROASTED NUT MIX

546. SWEET AND SOUR DRY ROASTED NUT MIX

547. LEMON AND CAYANNE DRY ROASTED NUT MIX

548. LEMON AND CAJUN DRY ROASTED NUT MIX

549. LEMON AND HAVENERO DRY ROASTED NUT MIX

550. LEMON AND ONION DRY ROASTED NUT MIX

551. LEMON AND GARLIC DRY ROASTED NUT MIX

552. NECTURINE ICE CREAM

553. SPICE ICE CREAM

554. THIN CORN BREAD

555. NECTURINE CREAM PIE

556. CINNAMON PIE

557. CINNAMON CHEESE CAKE

558. CINNAMON DATE PASTRY

559. CARMELIZED CINNAMON TART

560. CINNAMON CANDY

561. LICORICE ICE CREAM

562. LICORICE FROSTING

563. LICORICE BAKED ALASKA

564. LICORICE CHEESE CAKE

565. LICORICE TOFFEE COOKIES

566. LICORICE FUDGE

567. LICORICE SALT WATER TOFFEE

568. LICORICE COCONUT CARMELS
569. LICORICE CANDY
570. LICORICE COCONUT COOKIES
571. LICORICE MACROONS
572. HAVANERO RICE
573. MARTIN MASSOOD TAIS LICORICE SANDWICH COOKIES
574. CINNAMON SANDWICH COOKIES
575. CORN ON THE COB
576. AVA DANIELLE NEUMILLER ORANGE CREAM PIE
577. CINNAMON WALNUT FUDGE
578. WALNUT CRUST FOR ANY PIE
579. GREEN PEAS AND RICE
580. LEMON CREAM PIE
581. COCONUT CREAM PIE
582. PUMPKIN AND APPLE COOKIES
583. SUCANANT FACE COOKIES
584. HAZEL NUT FACE COOKIES
585. HAZEL NUT CAROB COOKIES
586. PISTACHIO FACE COOKIES
587. PISTACHIO AND CASHEW COOKIES
588. PERO SUCANANT COOKIES
589. HAZELNUT SPICE COOKIES
590. CINNAMON WALNUT FACE COOKIES
591. CAROB-COCONUT FACE COOKIES
592. LEMON WALNUT COOKIES
593. ORANGE WALNUT COOKIES
594. ANISE WALNUT COOKIES
595. PEPPERMINT WALNUT COOKIES
596. CAROB COCONUT PIE COOKIES
597. PERO AND HAZELNUT PIE COOKIES
598. CARMELIZED CINNAMON PISTACHIO TART
599. VITAMIX LICORICE MACROONS
600. VITAMIX CINNAMON MACROONS
601. VITAMIX PEPPERMINT MACROONS
602. WIN TINSON STRAWBERRY CREAM PIE
603. STRAWBERRY ICE CREAM

604. STRAWBERRY CHEESE CAKE
605. BLUEBERRY CHEESE CAKE
606. STRAWBERRY BAKED ALASKA
607. STRAWBERRY MAPLE CAKE
608. STRAWBERRY UPSIDE DOWN CREAM CAKE
609. FIRE DRY ROASTED NUT MIX
610. CITRUS AND HERB RICE
611. BAR-B-QUE SEASONED RICE
612. MEXICAN SEASONED RICE
613. JAMAICAN SEASONED RICE
614. ITALIAN SEASONED RICE
615. TACO SEASONED RICE
616. THAI SEASONED RICE
617. PIZZA SEASONED RICE
618. CAJUN SEASONED RICE
619. ORIENTAL SEASONED RICE
620. CAROB CASHEW CREAM PIE
621. PERO CASHEW CREAM PIE
622. CINNAMON CASHEW CREAM PIE
623. LEMON CASHEW CREAM PIE
624. ORANGE CASHEW CREAM PIE
625. SPICE CASHEW CREAM PIE
626. LICORICE AND CASHEW CREAM PIE
627. GREEN HOT SAUCE
628. GREEN SALSA
629. SESAME SEED BISCUITS
630. ITALIAN BISCUITS
631. GARLIC BISCUITS
632. HOT BISCUITS
633. SOYMILK BISCUITS
634. POPPY SEED BISCUITS
635. HUNZA BREAD

CONCLUSION

This book illustrates just why coffee, chocolate, teas, and sodas should be eliminated immediately, and replaced! There is no excuse to continue to consume them, especially since there are recipes that replace all junk foods. These delicious foods will not harm your body and cause a host of other problems now and later. The added chemicals and over processing combined is enough reasons for them to be replaced. The bad coffee, chocolate, teas, also have insect fragments, and rodent hairs, which do not help your body. This book makes it obvious coffee, chocolate, teas, and sodas must be replaced!

REFERENCES

Dr Ede Koenig

Aileen Ludingtom MD

Dr Agatha Thrash